The Concise Book of Yoga Anatomy

An Illustrated Guide to the Science of Motion

Jo Ann Staugaard-Jones

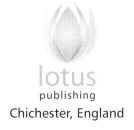

lotus
publishing
Chichester, England

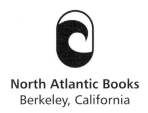

North Atlantic Books
Berkeley, California

First published in 2015 by
Lotus Publishing
Apple Tree Cottage, Inlands Road, Nutbourne, Chichester, PO18 8RJ and
North Atlantic Books
Berkeley, California

All Drawings Amanda Williams
Text Design Wendy Craig
Cover Design Jasmine Hromjak
Printed and Bound in the UK by Bell and Bain Limited

The Concise Book of Yoga Anatomy: An Illustrated Guide to the Science of Motion is sponsored and published by the Society for the Study of Native Arts and Sciences (dba North Atlantic Books), an educational nonprofit based in Berkeley, California, that collaborates with partners to develop cross-cultural perspectives, nurture holistic views of art, science, the humanities, and healing, and seed personal and global transformation by publishing work on the relationship of body, spirit, and nature.

North Atlantic Books' publications are available through most bookstores. For further information, visit our website at www.northatlanticbooks .com or call 800-733-3000.

Disclaimer: This book offers health and movement information and is for educational purposes only. It is not a substitute for, nor does it replace, professional medical advice, diagnosis or treatment of health conditions.

British Library Cataloguing-in-Publication Data
A CIP record for this book is available from the British Library
ISBN 978 1 905367 56 6 (Lotus Publishing)
ISBN 978 1 58394 983 2 (North Atlantic Books)

Library of Congress Cataloging-in-Publication Data
Staugaard-Jones, Jo Ann, author.
The concise book of yoga anatomy : an illustrated guide to the science of motion / Jo Ann Staugaard-Jones.
    p. ; cm.
Includes bibliographical references and indexes.
ISBN 978-1-58394-983-2 (pbk.) — ISBN 978-1-58394-984-9 (ebook)
I. Title.
[DNLM: 1. Yoga. 2. Kinesiology, Applied. 3. Muscles—physiology. QT 260.5.Y7]
RA781.7
613.7'046—dc23
                     2015013328

Contents

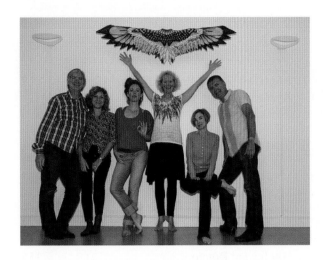

Thank you, Paris models and Atelier Marais Studio!
From left to right:

Reinhard Fleer, Paris, France; Molecular Biologist, Amateur Photographer.
reinhard.fleer@gmail.com

Claire Bertin, born and raised in Paris, France; French and Comparative Literature teacher, writer.

Ingy Ganga, from France, Egypt, and Turkey; Yin/Hatha Yoga teacher and soul singer in Paris.
www.ingyganga.in

Jo Ann Staugaard-Jones, Cranberry Lake, NJ; Author, Yoga Anatomy Teacher Trainer.
www.move-live.com

Jo Ann Hegre, an American who has lived in Paris for 25 years; Geologist; spends her time hiking and biking; an ex-dancer who now does yoga.

René Montaz-Rosset, Paris, France; Engineer; spends his time hiking, biking, skiing; started doing yoga in 2011.

All photo shooting on the premises of:

**Atelier Marais
54, rue Charlot
75003 Paris**
http://www.atelier-marais.fr
http://www.b-y-p.be

About this Book

This book is designed in quick-reference format to offer useful information about the main skeletal muscles that are central to yoga. It is my belief that yoga styles that include the limb of yoga called *asana*[1] (which has evolved to become a term that signifies all yoga postures) should be taught and practiced in a way that is comfortable, stable, balanced, and without pain. Understanding the science of the body and of motion will help one to achieve this.

To assist your understanding of the biomechanics of the body, each muscle section is color-coded for ease of reference. Enough detail is included regarding the muscle's origin, insertion, and action to meet the requirements of the student, practitioner, and teacher of all yoga movement. The book aims to present that information accurately, in a clear and user-friendly format, especially as anatomy and kinesiology can seem heavily laden with terminology. Technical terms are therefore explained throughout the text.

Major muscles are identified and asana illustrations help to show how they are working in relation to the particular posture. Each asana is listed in Sanskrit (phonetically, with definition) and English, with sections to describe awareness, joint actions, alignment, technique, helpful hints, and counter poses (postures that are helpful to counteract the illustrated asana). Knowledge of all this is paramount to the ability to teach or practice with no injury to oneself or to others. As mechanics are emphasized and learned, I ask that you take the time to then realize the *essence* of the pose or movement in relation to the yogic way of life, for it is necessary to focus on the spiritual element of yoga as well as the physical. Yoga is a union of the two, so where appropriate, the more profound side of the practice is mentioned as it relates to the body.

As an example, when one sits in meditation in *Sukhasana* (Easy Pose), the postural aspects can be the beginning of the process, but as breathing and subtle energies are incorporated, the fundamental nature might be the stillness of the mind in order to reach inner awareness. Explore each posture and consider more deeply what the asana means for you.

In what is termed *Hatha Yoga* (the foundational form represented in this book), the sun and the moon represent the two polar energies of the human body. The word *hatha* itself, divided into syllables of "ha" and "tha," suggests the solar and lunar energies. *Atha* is also defined as now, *yoga* as union, balance.

When faced with the choice of what yoga style to study, I chose one with strong tradition and science interwoven. Hatha yoga provides the all-important deep breath work, support, strength, flexibility, and progression needed to lead one to a well-balanced and profound practice. Attention is given not only to the gross anatomy stated in this book, but the subtle yet powerful physical and energetic forces of the body as well.

Thus, asana can lead one to going inward, with effortless breath, stillness, and meditation, as "complete mastery over the roaming tendencies of the mind is Yoga." (Tigunait, 2014)

In *The Concise Book of Yoga Anatomy* you will not find the asanas categorized under type, such as "Standing", but placed under a specific muscle that is used in that posture. It is yet another way to look at the anatomy of yoga.

As students, guides, and facilitators of yoga, and as human beings looking to understand the physical, mental, and spiritual aspects, we can use yoga as a blueprint toward the study of form and the philosophy of living: "do no harm" (in Sanskrit, *ahimsa*).

People do yoga for many reasons; whatever the basis, yoga is always a path to truth. This can be blocked if there is pain. My contribution in teaching Yoga Anatomy and Kinesiology is to help people be free from injury in asanas, and to become less mechanical and more aware, open, and able to move toward their own true selves.

Jo Ann Staugaard-Jones www.move-live.com

---

[1]   Asanas are one of Patanjali's Eight Limbs of Yoga.

1

The Moving Body

Guide to the Nervous System

The human nervous system controls the functions of each different system of the body by means of neurons. It has two parts:

1. Central nervous system (CNS): encompasses the brain and spinal cord. This system enables us to think, learn, reason, and maintain balance.

2. Peripheral nervous system (PNS): located outside the brain and spinal cord, in the outer parts of the body. This system helps us to carry out voluntary and involuntary actions and enables feeling through the senses.

The PNS comprises the following:

1. Autonomic nervous system (ANS): responsible for regulating the internal organs and glands; it controls involuntary actions. The ANS consists of three subsystems:

    ι.   Sympathetic nervous system: activates what is commonly known as the "fight or flight" response.
    ιι. Parasympathetic nervous system: stimulates what are referred to as "rest and digest" activities.
    ιιι. Enteric nervous system: controls the gastrointestinal system in vertebrates.

2. Somatic nervous system (SNS): carries information from nerves to the CNS and from the CNS to the muscles and sensory fibers; it is associated with voluntary muscle control.

The practice of somatics is noted in this book as, quite simply, using the body's intelligence. The integration of the mind, body, and feelings to allow the body's non-verbal communication system to respond in a healthy way is key to wellness. Somatic healing is about getting in touch with the "sixth sense" (intuitive response) to facilitate a breakthrough in personal health. It is about listening to a language of immediate experiences. Kinesthetic awareness is part of this: being present, listening to the body, and being conscious and knowledgeable about where our bodies are in space and what is happening anatomically is paramount to yoga. A well-balanced, continual yoga practice leads to muscle memory and intelligence through nerve impulse as well. The nervous system is extremely complex. Try to follow the pathway of just one nerve, the genitofemoral. This nerve

*   is part of the upper region of the lumbar plexus, one of three components of the larger lumbosacral plexus of the lower vertebral column;
*   originates from L1 and L2 nerve roots;
*   emerges on the anterior surface of the psoas major muscle, where the lumbar plexus is embedded and has many branches;
*   divides into a femoral branch and a genital branch;
*   supplies the skin anterior to the upper part of the femoral triangle;
*   in males, travels through the inguinal canal, supplying the cremaster muscle (covering the testes) and scrotal skin;
*   in females, ends in the skin of the mons pubis (anterior portion of the vulva) and the labia majora. The function of these branches of the genitofemoral nerve is sensory in both genders.

Relationship Between Different Parts of the Nervous System

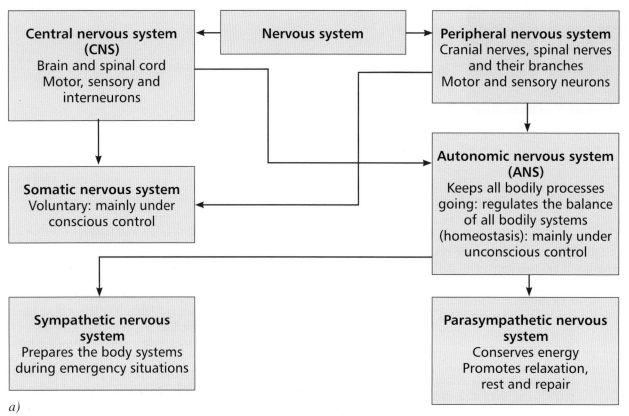

a)

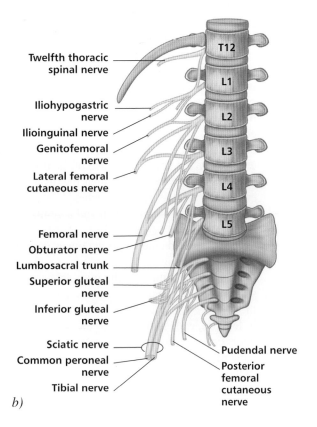

Twelfth thoracic
spinal nerve

Iliohypogastric
nerve

Ilioinguinal nerve

Genitofemoral
nerve

Lateral femoral
cutaneous nerve

Femoral nerve

Obturator nerve

Lumbosacral trunk

Superior gluteal
nerve

Inferior gluteal
nerve

Sciatic nerve

Common peroneal
nerve

Tibial nerve

T12
L1
L2
L3
L4
L5

Pudendal nerve

Posterior
femoral
cutaneous
nerve

b)

This information is included to prove how difficult it is to deal with neurology in yoga. However, the nerve complex can be referred to if one has the knowledge to do so.

Nerve Entrapment
Nerve entrapment is compression that may become a source of pain and can be reduced if practicing the correct asanas. (The expression "pinched nerve" usually refers to carpal tunnel syndrome or sciatica, but it is applicable to any pressure on a particular nerve or group of nerves.) As an example, when a person experiences sciatica, it is usually indicated by pain along the path of the sciatic nerve from the spine into the posterior thigh. A common muscle that can trap this nerve is the piriformis (Chapter 8). A yoga practitioner can use any number of stretches or postures (such as a supine twist) to relax this muscle, thus lessening the pressure on the sciatic nerve that passes behind it.

Figure 1.1: a) Nervous system table;
b) Genitofemoral nerve.

Another example of nerve impingement that might be relieved by yoga is in the brachial plexus area. This is a network of nerves that sends signals from the spine to the shoulder, arm, and hand. A brachial plexus injury occurs when these nerves are stretched, pinched, or even torn (this would require surgery). This area is compromised if the posture of the neck or shoulders (such as rounding) interferes with the path of a nerve impulse. Any yoga posture that emphasizes spine extension and shoulder placement (typically "back and down")—for example Mountain Pose (*Tadasana*)—will help to open this area.

Causes are specific to the area of concern and can range from degenerating discs, bone spurs, arthritis, and muscle dysfunction to injury and emotional trauma causing muscle tension. It is best to have a licensed therapist, physician, or neurologist diagnose the condition.

It has been proven that nerve entrapment may be relieved through muscular release. Some asanas can do this.

A Note About Peripheral Nerve Supply

The relevant peripheral nerve supply is listed with each muscle presented in this book, for those who want to know. However, information about the spinal segment[2] from which the nerve fibers emanate often differs among sources. This is because it is extremely difficult for anatomists to trace the route of an individual nerve fiber through the intertwining maze of other nerve fibers as it passes through its plexus (plexus = a network of nerves: from the Latin word *plectere*, meaning "to braid"). The most applicable nerve roots for each muscle have been adopted for this book.

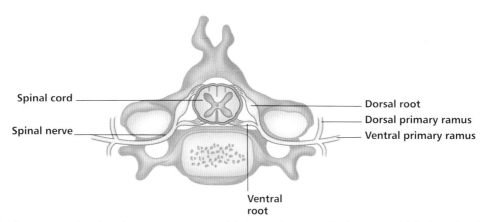

Spinal cord — Dorsal root — Dorsal primary ramus — Ventral primary ramus — Spinal nerve — Ventral root

Figure 1.2: A spinal segment showing the nerve roots combining to form a spinal nerve, which then divides into ventral and dorsal rami.

2   A spinal segment is the part of the spinal cord that gives rise to each pair of spinal nerves (a pair consists of one nerve for the left side of the body and one for the right side). Each spinal nerve contains motor and sensory fibers. Soon after the spinal nerve exits through the foramen (the opening between adjacent vertebrae), it divides into a dorsal primary ramus (directed posteriorly) and a ventral primary ramus (directed laterally or anteriorly). Fibers from the dorsal rami innervate the skin and extensor muscles of the neck and trunk. The ventral rami supply the limbs, in addition to the sides and front of the trunk.

Anatomical Orientation

Anatomical Directions

To describe the relative positions of body parts and their movements, it is essential to have a universally accepted reference position. The standard body position, known as the "anatomical position," serves as this reference. Anatomical position is simply standing upright with arms hanging by the sides, palms facing forward (see Figure 1.3). Most directional terminology used refers to the body as if it were in the anatomical position, regardless of its actual position. Note also that the terms "left" and "right" refer to the sides of the object or person being viewed and not those of the reader.

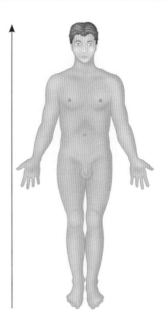

*Figure 1.5: **Superior***
Above; toward the head or upper part of the structure or body.

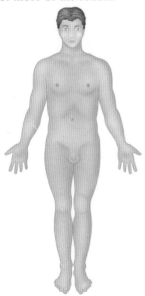

*Figure 1.3: **Anterior***
In front of; toward or at the front of the body.

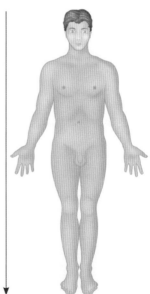

*Figure 1.6: **Inferior***
Below; away from the head or toward the lower part of the structure or body.

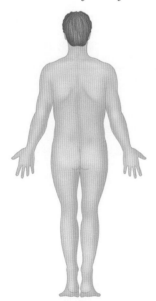

*Figure 1.4: **Posterior***
Behind; toward or at the back of the body.

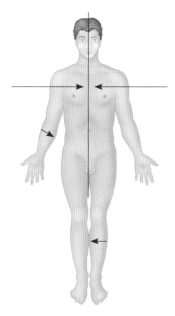

Figure 1.7: **Medial**
(From medius in Latin, meaning "middle")
Toward or at the midline of the body; on the inner side of a limb.

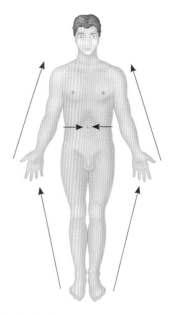

Figure 1.9: **Proximal**
(From proximus in Latin, meaning "nearest")
Closer to the center of the body (the navel) or to the attachment point of a limb to the torso.

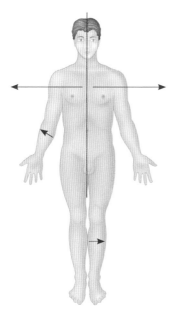

Figure 1.8: **Lateral**
(From latus in Latin, meaning "side")
Away from the midline of the body; on the outer side of the body or a limb.

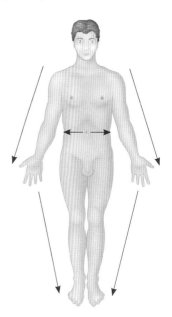

Figure 1.10: **Distal**
(From distans in Latin, meaning "distant")
Farther away from the center of the body, or from the attachment point of a limb to the torso.

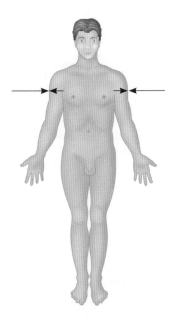

Figure 1.11: **Superficial**
Toward or at the body surface.

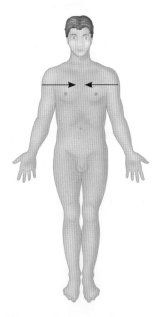

Figure 1.12: **Deep**
Farther away from the body surface; more internal.

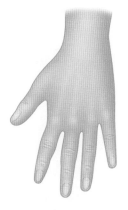

Figure 1.13: **Dorsal**
The posterior surface of something, e.g., the back of the hand or top of the foot.

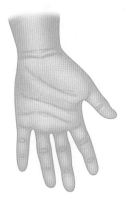

Figure 1.14: **Palmar**
The anterior surface of the hand, i.e., the palm.

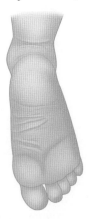

Figure 1.15: **Plantar**
The sole of the foot.

Planes of the Body

The term "planes" refers to two-dimensional sections through the body. They provide a view of the body or body part, as though it has been cut through by an imaginary line.

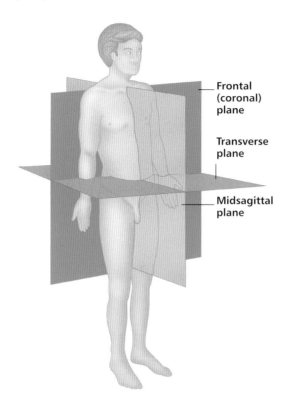

Figure 1.16: Planes of the body.

- The sagittal planes cut vertically through the body from anterior to posterior, dividing it into right and left halves. Figure 1.16 shows the midsagittal plane.
- The frontal (coronal) planes pass vertically through the body, dividing it into anterior and posterior sections, and lie at right angles to the sagittal plane.
- The transverse planes are horizontal cross-sections, dividing the body into upper (superior) and lower (inferior) sections, and lie at right angles to the other two planes. Figure 1.16 illustrates the most frequently used planes.

Use of the three major planes is important in yoga because the body is meant to work in all planes in order for it to be most efficient. When one practices yoga in a structured class, it is wise to incorporate movement in all planes by using various asanas. Examples are as follows:

SAGITTAL: **Sun Salutation** (*Surya Namaska*); (*surya* = sun; *namaskar* = salute)

1. Begin in **Mountain Pose**.
2. Inhale to **Crescent Stretch**: bring the arms overhead and stretch to the sky.
3. Exhale and release to **Forward Bend**.
4. Inhale, lifting the spine forward to an extended position, with hands on the shins.
5. Exhale to **Forward Bend**.
6. Inhale and take one leg back to a **lunge** position.
7. Exhale and take the other leg back to **Plank** and lower to the floor.
8. Inhale to **Cobra**.
9. Exhale to **Child's Pose**. Rest for three full breaths.
10. Inhale to **Table** position.
11. Exhale to **Down Dog**. Rest for three long, full *Ujjayi* (Ocean Breaths).
12. Inhale, walking or jumping the feet to a position between the hands.
13. Exhale to **Forward Bend**. Inhale and do number 4, then exhale back to **Forward Bend**.
14. Inhale to roll up the spine, raising the arms to the sky (**Reverse Swan Dive**).
15. Exhale to **Mountain Pose** (hands in *Namaste*, prayer position, centering and sealing the practice).

FRONTAL: Gate Pose (*Parighasana*) or any posture that incorporates abduction or adduction of a particular joint, or lateral flexion of the spine (side bending).

HORIZONTAL: Revolved Triangle (*Parivrtta Trikonasana*) or any spinal twist or rotary movements, such as supination/pronation.

Anatomical Movements

The direction in which body parts move is described in relation to the fetal position. Moving into the fetal position results from flexion of all the limbs. Straightening out of the fetal position results from extension of all the limbs. These actions are also done in the sagittal plane.

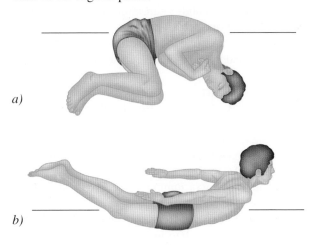

a)

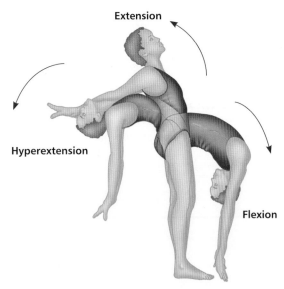

b)

Figure 1.17: a) Flexion into the fetal position;
b) Extension out of the fetal position.

Main Movements

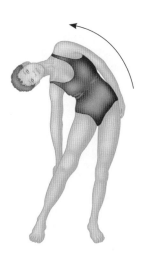

*Figure 1.19: **Lateral Flexion:** Bending the torso or head laterally (sideways) in the frontal (coronal) plane.*

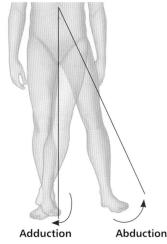

Adduction   Abduction

*Figure 20: **Abduction:** Movement of a bone away from the midline of the body or the midline of a limb.*
***Adduction:** Movement of a bone toward the midline of the body or the midline of a limb.*

*Figure 1.18: **Flexion:** Bending to decrease the angle between bones at a joint. From the anatomical position, flexion is usually forward, except at the knee joint, where it is backward. The way to remember this is that flexion is always toward the fetal position.*
***Extension:** Straightening or bending backward away from the fetal position.*
***Hyperextension:** Extending the limb beyond its normal range of motion.*

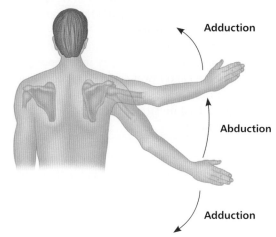

Adduction

Abduction

Adduction

Note: For abduction of the arm to continue above the height of the shoulder (elevation through abduction, see p. 16), the scapula must rotate on its axis to turn the glenoid cavity upward (see Figure 1.28b).

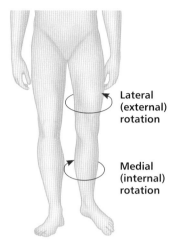

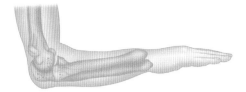

Figure 1.23: a) **Pronation:** *To turn the palm of the hand down to face the floor (if standing with elbow bent to 90°, or if lying flat on the floor) or away from the anatomical and fetal positions.*

Figure 1.21: **Rotation:** *Movement of a bone or the trunk around its own longitudinal axis.*
Medial rotation: *To turn in, toward the midline.*
Lateral rotation: *To turn out, away from the midline.*

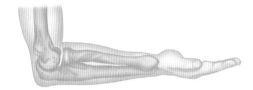

Figure 1.23: b) **Supination:** *To turn the palm of the hand up to face the ceiling (if standing with elbow bent to 90°, or if lying flat on the floor) or toward the anatomical and fetal positions.*

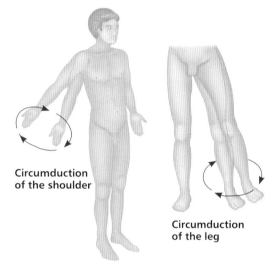

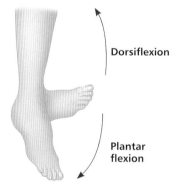

Figure 1.22: **Circumduction:** *Movement in which the distal end of a bone moves in a circle, while the proximal end remains stable; it is a combination of flexion, abduction, extension, and adduction.*

Figure 1.24: **Plantar flexion:** *To point the toes down toward the ground.*
Dorsiflexion: *To point the toes toward the sky (a popular yoga position).*

Other Movements

The movements given in this section are those that occur only at specific joints or parts of the body, usually involving more than one joint.

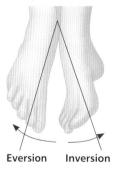

Figure 1.25: **Inversion:** *To turn the sole of the foot inward, so that the soles would face each other; weight would be on the outside of the foot (sometimes referred to as "supination").*
Eversion: *To turn the sole of the foot outward, so that the soles would face away from each other; weight would be on the inside of the foot (sometimes referred to as "pronation").*

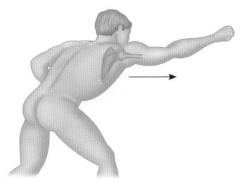

Figure 1.26: **Protraction:** *Movement forward in the transverse plane. For example, protracting the shoulder girdle, as in rounding the shoulder.*

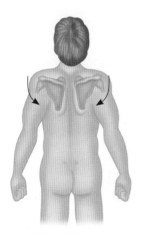

Figure 1.27: **Retraction:** *Movement backward in the transverse plane, as in bracing the shoulder girdle back, military style.*

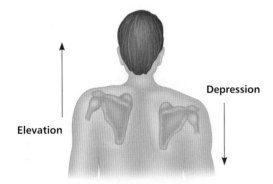

Figure 1.28: a) **Elevation:** *Movement of a part of the body upward along the frontal plane. For example, elevating the scapula by shrugging the shoulders.* **Depression:** *Movement of an elevated part of the body downward to its original position.*

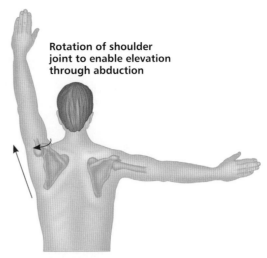

Rotation of shoulder joint to enable elevation through abduction

Figure 1.28: b) Abducting the arm at the shoulder joint, then continuing to raise it above the head in the frontal plane can be referred to as **"elevation through abduction."** *In yoga, as the arms are raised overhead, the action of depressing the shoulder girdle is emphasized once the full position is reached, as in Warrior I or Down Dog.*

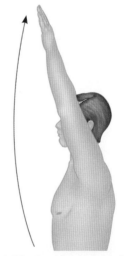

Figure 1.28: c) Flexing the arm at the shoulder joint, then continuing to raise it above the head in the sagittal plane can be referred to as **"elevation through flexion."**

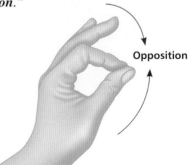

Opposition

Figure 1.29: **Opposition:** *Movement specific to the saddle joint of the human thumb, which enables one to touch the thumb to the tip of each finger of the same hand.*

Skeletal System

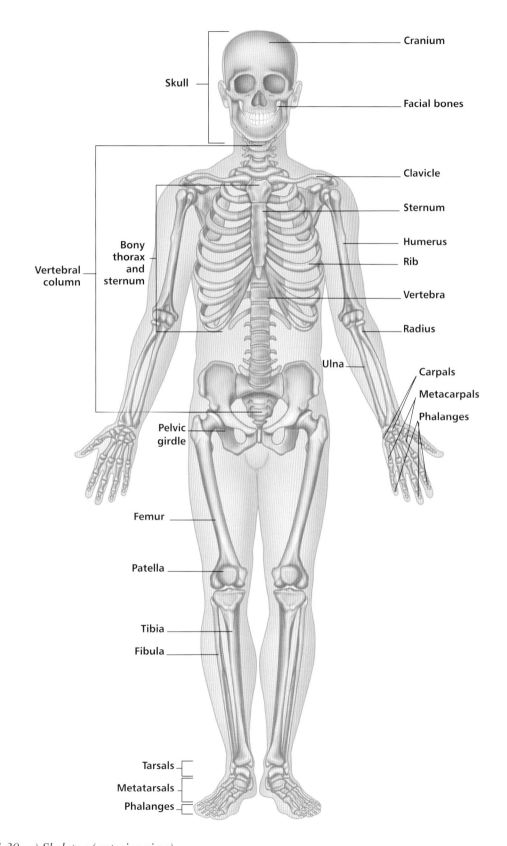

Figure 1.30: a) Skeleton (anterior view).

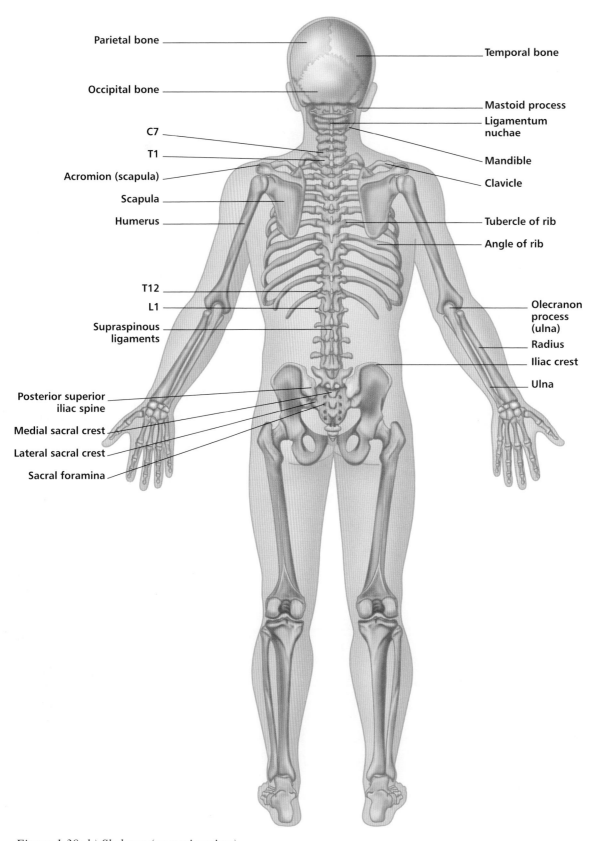

Parietal bone

Occipital bone

C7

T1

Acromion (scapula)

Scapula

Humerus

T12

L1

Supraspinous
ligaments

Posterior superior
iliac spine

Medial sacral crest

Lateral sacral crest

Sacral foramina

Temporal bone

Mastoid process

Ligamentum
nuchae

Mandible

Clavicle

Tubercle of rib

Angle of rib

Olecranon
process
(ulna)

Radius

Iliac crest

Ulna

Figure 1.30: b) Skeleton (posterior view).

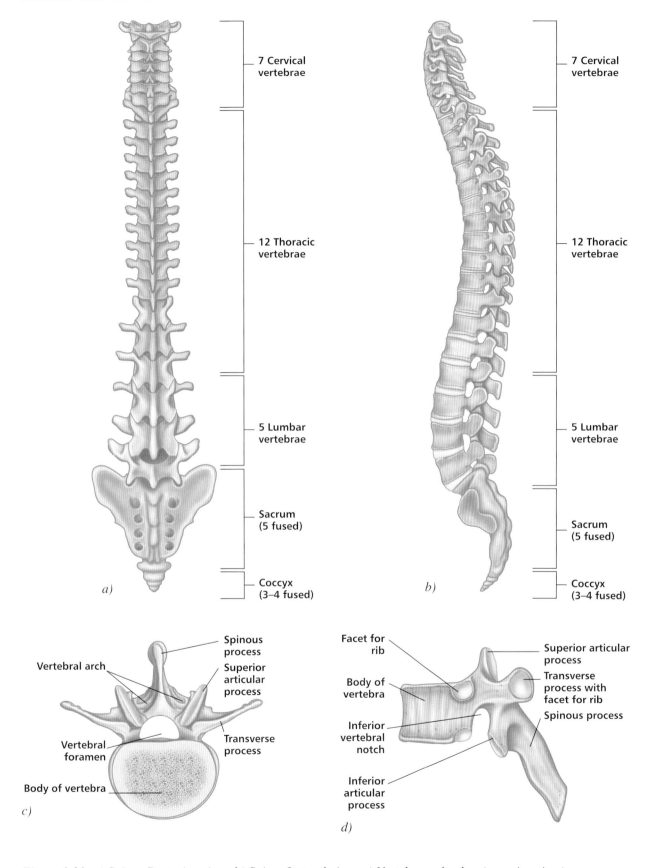

7 Cervical vertebrae

12 Thoracic vertebrae

5 Lumbar vertebrae

Sacrum (5 fused)

Coccyx (3–4 fused)

a)

7 Cervical vertebrae

12 Thoracic vertebrae

5 Lumbar vertebrae

Sacrum (5 fused)

Coccyx (3–4 fused)

b)

Spinous process

Superior articular process

Vertebral arch

Transverse process

Vertebral foramen

Body of vertebra

c)

Facet for rib

Superior articular process

Transverse process with facet for rib

Body of vertebra

Spinous process

Inferior vertebral notch

Inferior articular process

d)

Figure 1.31: a) Spine: Posterior view; b) Spine: Lateral view; c) Vertebrae — lumbar (superior view) and d) Thoracic (lateral view).

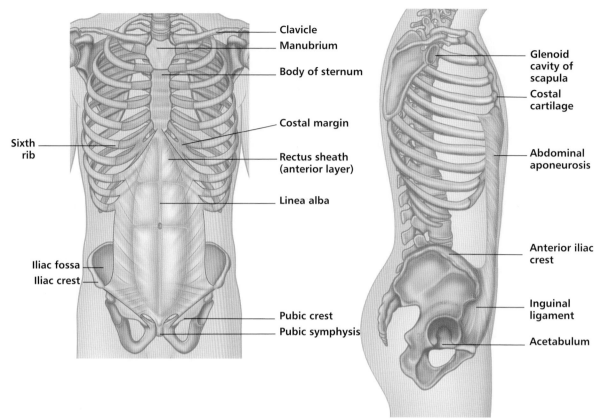

Clavicle
Manubrium
Body of sternum
Costal margin
Rectus sheath (anterior layer)
Linea alba
Sixth rib
Iliac fossa
Iliac crest
Pubic crest
Pubic symphysis

Glenoid cavity of scapula
Costal cartilage
Abdominal aponeurosis
Anterior iliac crest
Inguinal ligament
Acetabulum

Figure 1.32: a) Anterior view; b) Lateral view.

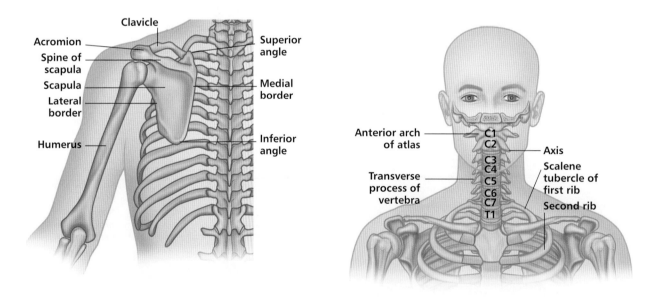

Clavicle
Acromion
Spine of scapula
Scapula
Lateral border
Humerus
Superior angle
Medial border
Inferior angle

Anterior arch of atlas
Transverse process of vertebra
C1
C2
C3
C4
C5
C6
C7
T1
Axis
Scalene tubercle of first rib
Second rib

Figure 1.33: Scapula (posterior view).

Figure 1.34: Skull to sternum (anterior view—the mandible and maxilla are removed).

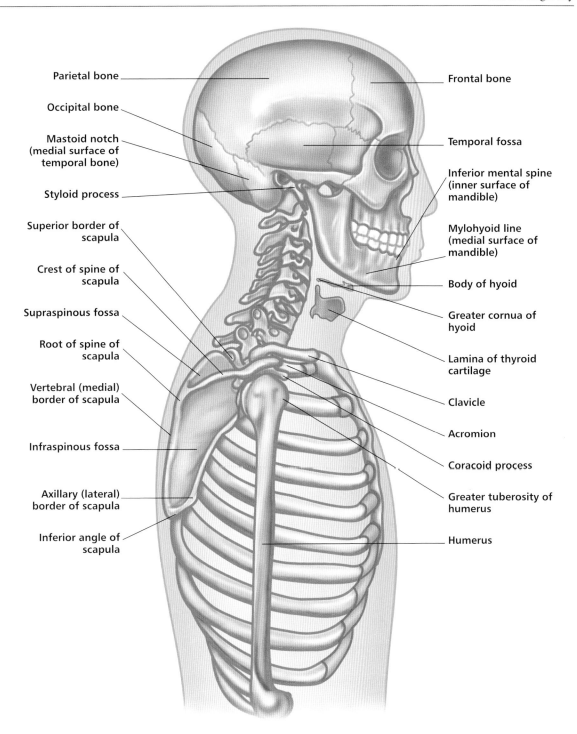

Parietal bone

Frontal bone

Occipital bone

Mastoid notch
(medial surface of
temporal bone)

Temporal fossa

Inferior mental spine
(inner surface of
mandible)

Styloid process

Superior border of
scapula

Mylohyoid line
(medial surface of
mandible)

Crest of spine of
scapula

Body of hyoid

Supraspinous fossa

Greater cornua of
hyoid

Root of spine of
scapula

Lamina of thyroid
cartilage

Vertebral (medial)
border of scapula

Clavicle

Infraspinous fossa

Acromion

Coracoid process

Axillary (lateral)
border of scapula

Greater tuberosity of
humerus

Inferior angle of
scapula

Humerus

Figure 1.35: Skull to humerus (lateral view).

Synovial Joints

Joints, or articulations, have two functions: they provide stability and give the rigid skeleton mobility. Immovable (synarthrotic) and slightly movable (amphiarthrotic) joints are found mainly in the axial skeleton, where joint stability is important to protect the internal organs. Synovial joints are freely movable (diarthrotic), and so are found predominately in the limbs, where a greater range of movement is required. These joints have a number of distinguishing features:

- Articular (hyaline) cartilage covering the ends of the bones that form the joint
- A joint cavity filled with lubricating synovial fluid (a slippery fluid which provides a film that reduces friction)
- Collateral or accessory ligaments that provide reinforcement and strength
- Bursae (fluid-filled sacs) that provide cushioning
- Tendon sheaths which wrap themselves around tendons that are subject to friction, in order to protect them

Articular discs (menisci) are present in some synovial joints (e.g., the knee) and act as shock absorbers. There are six types of synovial joint: plane (or gliding), hinge, pivot, ball-and-socket, condyloid, and saddle.

Plane or Gliding
Movement occurs when two generally flat or slightly curved surfaces glide across one another. Examples include the acromioclavicular and sacroiliac joints.

Hinge
Movement occurs around only one axis, a transverse one, as in the hinge of the lid of a box. A protrusion of one bone fits into a concave or cylindrical articular surface of another, permitting flexion and extension. Examples include the interphalangeal joints, the elbow, and the knee.

Pivot
Movement takes place around a vertical axis, like the hinge of a gate. A more or less cylindrical articular surface of bone protrudes into and rotates within a ring formed by bone or ligament. An example is the joint between the radius and the ulna at the elbow.

Ball-and-Socket
This joint consists of a "ball" formed by the spherical or hemispherical head of one bone that rotates within the concave "socket" of another, allowing flexion, extension, adduction, abduction, circumduction, and rotation. Thus these joints are multiaxial and allow the greatest range of movement of all the joints. Examples are the shoulder and hip joints.

Condyloid
These joints have a spherical articular surface that fits into a matching concavity. They permit flexion, extension, abduction, and adduction; a combination of these is called "circumduction." Examples are the wrist and the metacarpophalangeal joints of the fingers (but not the thumb).

Saddle
In a saddle joint the two articulating surfaces respectively have convex and concave areas, which fit together like a saddle and a horse's back. Saddle joints permit even more movement than condyloid joints. An example is the carpometacarpal joint of the thumb, which allows opposition of the thumb to the fingers.

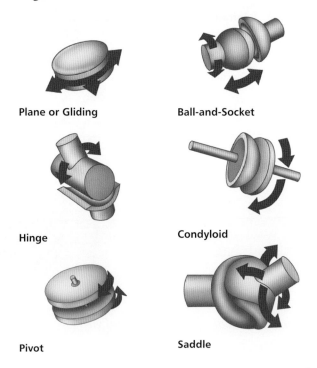

Plane or Gliding   Ball-and-Socket

Hinge   Condyloid

Pivot   Saddle

Figure 1.36: The synovial joints.

Guide to the Muscular System

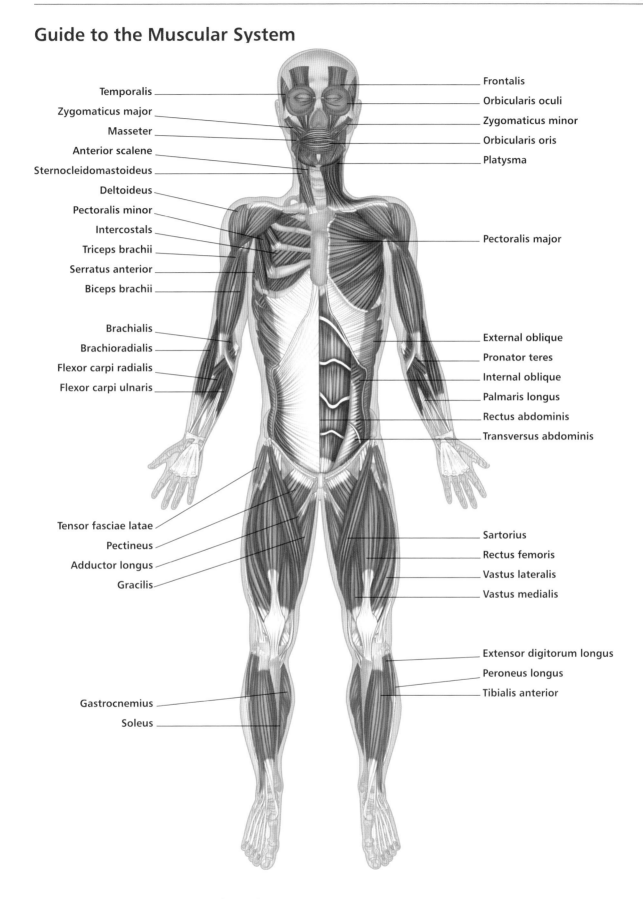

Temporalis

Zygomaticus major

Masseter

Anterior scalene

Sternocleidomastoideus

Deltoideus

Pectoralis minor

Intercostals

Triceps brachii

Serratus anterior

Biceps brachii

Brachialis

Brachioradialis

Flexor carpi radialis

Flexor carpi ulnaris

Tensor fasciae latae

Pectineus

Adductor longus

Gracilis

Gastrocnemius

Soleus

Frontalis

Orbicularis oculi

Zygomaticus minor

Orbicularis oris

Platysma

Pectoralis major

External oblique

Pronator teres

Internal oblique

Palmaris longus

Rectus abdominis

Transversus abdominis

Sartorius

Rectus femoris

Vastus lateralis

Vastus medialis

Extensor digitorum longus

Peroneus longus

Tibialis anterior

Figure 1.37: a) The major skeletal muscles (anterior view).

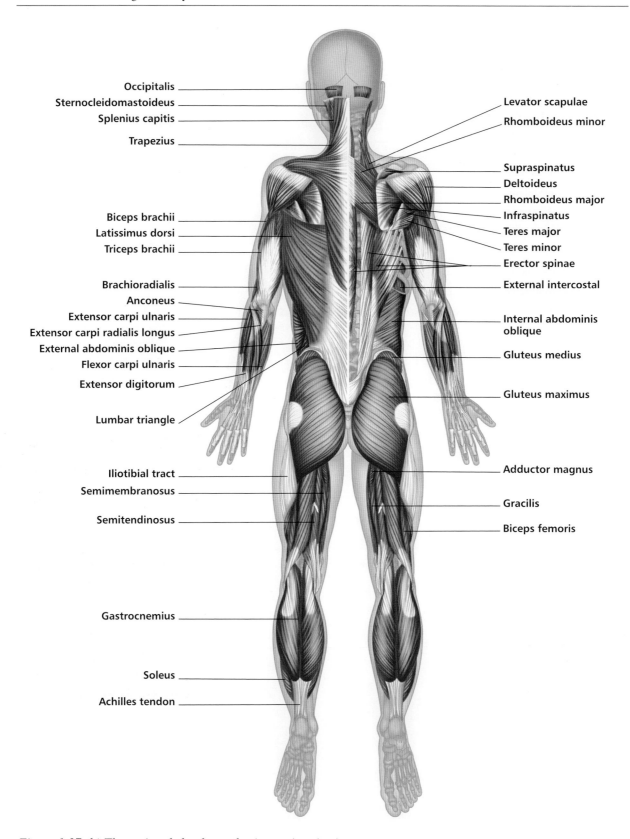

Occipitalis

Sternocleidomastoideus

Splenius capitis

Trapezius

Levator scapulae

Rhomboideus minor

Supraspinatus

Deltoideus

Rhomboideus major

Biceps brachii

Latissimus dorsi

Triceps brachii

Infraspinatus

Teres major

Teres minor

Erector spinae

Brachioradialis

Anconeus

Extensor carpi ulnaris

Extensor carpi radialis longus

External abdominis oblique

Flexor carpi ulnaris

Extensor digitorum

External intercostal

Internal abdominis oblique

Gluteus medius

Gluteus maximus

Lumbar triangle

Iliotibial tract

Semimembranosus

Semitendinosus

Adductor magnus

Gracilis

Biceps femoris

Gastrocnemius

Soleus

Achilles tendon

Figure 1.37: b) The major skeletal muscles (posterior view).

Muscle Attachment

Skeletal (somatic or voluntary) muscles constitute approximately 40% of the total human body weight. Their primary function is to produce movement by contracting and relaxing in a coordinated manner. They are attached to bone by tendons (or sometimes directly). The place where a muscle attaches to a relatively stationary point on a bone, either directly or via a tendon, is called the "origin." When the muscle contracts, it transmits tension to the bones across one or more joints, and movement occurs. The end of the muscle which attaches to the bone that moves is called the "insertion." Tendon attachments are also referred to as "proximal" (the one nearest the center) and "distal" (farthest from the center).

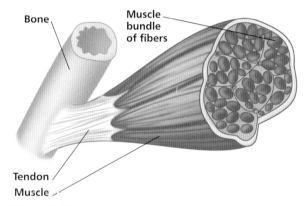

Figure 1.38: A tendon attachment.

Tendons and Aponeurosis

Muscle fascia (connective tissue components of a muscle) combine together and extend beyond the end of the muscle as round cords or flat bands called "tendons," or as a thin, flat, and broad sheet-like material called an "aponeurosis." The tendon or aponeurosis secures the muscle to the bone or cartilage, to other muscles, or to a seam of fibrous tissue called a "raphe" (a seam-like union of the two lateral halves of a part or organ, as in the tongue).

Intermuscular Septa

In some cases, flat sheets of dense connective tissue known as "intermuscular septa" penetrate between muscles, providing another medium to which muscle fibers may attach.

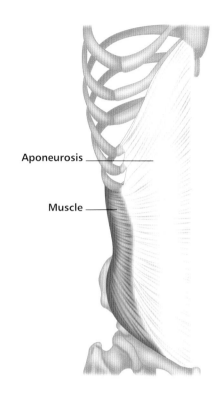

Figure 1.39: An attachment by aponeurosis.

Sesamoid Bones

If a tendon is subject to friction, it may (though not necessarily) develop a sesamoid bone within its substance. An example is the peroneus longus tendon in the sole of the foot. However, sesamoid bones might also appear in tendons not subject to friction. The main functions are to modify pressure, reduce friction, and sporadically change the direction of a muscle pull.

Multiple Attachments

Many muscles have only two attachments, one at each end. However, more complex muscles are often attached to several different structures at their origin and/or insertion. If these attachments are separated, effectively meaning the muscle gives rise to two or more tendons and/or aponeuroses inserting into different places, the muscle is said to have two heads. For example, the biceps brachii has two heads at its origin: one from the coracoid process of the scapula and one from the supraglenoid tubercle (see Chapter 6). The triceps brachii has three heads and the quadriceps has four.

Muscle Mechanics

A muscle will contract upon stimulation in an attempt to bring its attachments closer together, but this does not necessarily result in a shortening of the muscle. If the contraction of muscle results in the muscle creating movement of some sort, the contraction is called "isotonic"; if no movement results, the contraction is called "isometric."

Isometric Contraction

An isometric contraction occurs when a muscle increases its tension, but the length of the muscle is not altered. In other words, although the muscle tenses, the joint over which the muscle works does not move. One example of this is holding a heavy object in the hand with the elbow held stationary and bent at 90 degrees. Trying to lift something that proves to be too heavy to move is another example. Note also that some of the postural muscles are largely working isometrically by automatic reflex. For example, in the upright position, the body has a natural tendency to fall forward at the ankle. This is prevented by isometric contraction of the calf muscles. Likewise, the center of gravity of the skull would make the head tilt forward if the muscles at the back of the neck did not contract isometrically to keep it centralized. Isometric contractions are very common in yoga, as postures are held against an immovable force, such as the floor or a wall.

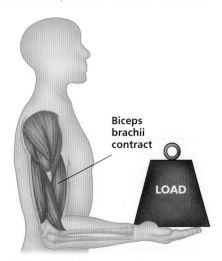

Figure 1.40: Isometric contraction.

Isotonic Contraction

Isotonic contractions of muscle enable us to move about. There are two types of isotonic contraction: "concentric" and "eccentric."

Concentric Contraction

In concentric contractions, the muscle attachments move closer together, causing movement at the joint. Using the example of holding an object, if the biceps brachii contracts concentrically, the elbow joint will flex and the hand will move toward the shoulder, against gravity. Similarly, if we do a sit-up exercise, the abdominal muscles contract concentrically to raise the torso.

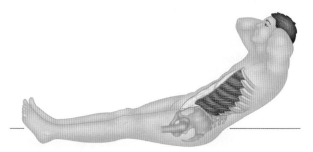

Figure 1.41: Abdominals contract concentrically to raise the body.

Eccentric Contraction

Eccentric contraction means that the muscle fibers "pay out" in a controlled manner to slow down movements in a case where gravity, if unchecked, would otherwise cause them to be too rapid—for example, lowering an object held in the hand down to your side. Another example is simply sitting down into a chair or lowering the torso after a sit-up exercise (the abdominals contract eccentrically to control the impact onto the floor). Therefore, the difference between concentric and eccentric contraction is that in the former, the muscle shortens, and in the latter, it lengthens.

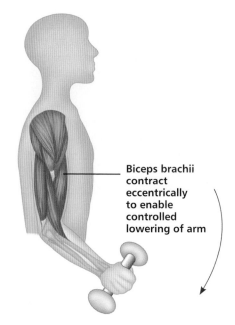

Figure 1.42: Eccentric isotonic contraction.

Group Action of Muscles

Muscles work together or in opposition to achieve a wide variety of movements. Therefore, whatever one muscle can do, there is another muscle that can undo it. Muscles may also be required to provide additional support or stability to enable certain movements to occur elsewhere.

Muscles are classified into four functional groups:

1. Prime mover or agonist
2. Antagonist
3. Synergist
4. Stabilizer

Prime Mover or Agonist

A prime mover (also called an "agonist") is a muscle that contracts to produce a specified movement. An example is the biceps brachii, which is the prime mover in elbow flexion. Other muscles may assist the prime mover in providing the same movement, albeit with less effect: such muscles are called "assistant movers" or "secondary movers." For example, the brachialis assists the biceps brachii in flexing the elbow and is therefore a secondary mover.

Antagonist

The muscle on the opposite side of a joint to the prime mover, and which must relax to allow the prime mover to contract, is called an "antagonist." For example, when the biceps brachii on the front of the arm contracts to flex the elbow, the triceps brachii on the back of the arm must relax to allow this movement to occur. When the movement is reversed, that is, when the elbow is extended against resistance, the triceps brachii becomes the prime mover and the biceps brachii assumes the role of antagonist.

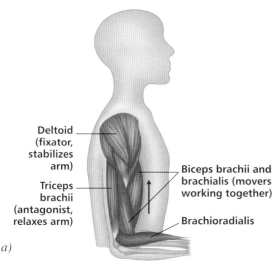

a)

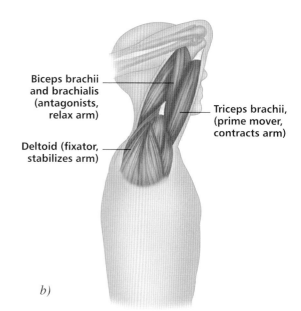

b)

Figure 1.43: Group action of muscles: a) Flexing the arm at the elbow; b) Extending the arm at the elbow (showing reversed roles of prime mover and antagonist).

Synergist

Synergists are muscles that enhance the movement of an agonist. They can also prevent any unwanted movements that might occur as the prime mover contracts. This is especially important where a prime mover crosses two joints, because when it contracts, it will cause movement at both joints, unless other muscles act to stabilize one of the joints. For example, the muscles that flex the fingers not only cross the finger joints, but also cross the wrist joint, potentially causing movement at both joints. However, because you have other muscles acting synergistically to stabilize the wrist joint, you are able to flex the fingers into a fist without also flexing the wrist at the same time.

A prime mover may have more than one action at the same or another joint, so synergists also act to eliminate the unwanted movements. For example, the biceps brachii will flex the elbow, but its line of pull will also supinate the forearm (twist the forearm, as in tightening a screw). If you want flexion to occur without supination, other muscles must contract to prevent this supination. In this context, such synergists are sometimes called "neutralizers," counterbalancing the unwanted movement.

Stabilizer

A synergist is more specifically referred to as a "fixator" or "stabilizer" when it immobilizes the bone of the prime mover's origin, thus providing a stable base for the action of the prime mover. The muscles that stabilize (fix) the scapula during movements of the upper limb are good examples. The sit-up exercise gives another good example. The abdominal muscles attach to both the rib cage and the pelvis. When they contract to enable you to perform a sit-up, the hip flexors will contract synergistically as fixators to prevent the abdominals from tilting the pelvis, thereby enabling the upper body to curl forward as the pelvis remains stationary.

Many yoga positions are held isometrically, against an immovable force such as the floor. This is a form of strength training. But to "get there and return from" a given position, muscles usually contract concentrically or eccentrically. To better understand these concepts, consider the following analysis of Boat Pose (*Navasana*).

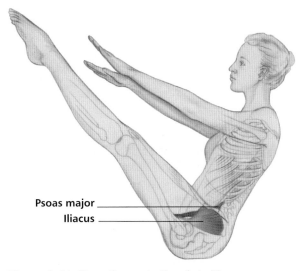

Psoas major _____
Iliacus _____

Figure 1.44: Boat Pose—in Sanskrit, Navasana.

Boat Pose (Figure 1.44) is mainly a hip flexion and spinal extension asana. If the arms are reaching forward, shoulder flexion is added.

Approach: The main muscles that are contracting concentrically (shortening) against resistance (gravity) "to get there" are the hip flexors: rectus femoris, sartorius, and iliopsoas. The hip adductors help to keep the legs together. The quadriceps muscles also contract to keep the knees straight. (If this pose is too challenging, the knees can bend and hands may be placed on the floor.)

If the pose is done correctly, the deep posterior muscles (transversalis, etc.) and other strong spine extensors (e.g., erector spinae) will also contract to straighten the spine against the resistance of gravity. Thus all the contracting muscles are the agonists (the movers, or mobilizers), and their antagonists are the muscles on the opposite side of the movers: the hip extensors (gluteus maximus and hamstrings), knee flexors (hamstrings), and spinal flexors (abdominals).

At the shoulder joint, the arm flexors (upper pectoralis major, anterior deltoid, biceps brachii, and coracobrachialis) are working to hold the arms forward in flexion against gravity.

Stabilizers: The psoas major is acting as a stabilizer for the hip and lumbar spine, and as a synergist with the iliacus in hip flexion. Other deep core muscles, such as the transversus abdominis and quadratus lumborum, are stabilizing the lower spine as well. The question is, what are the abdominals doing? One can certainly feel them working in this posture. The rectus abdominis and obliques are actually stabilizing, acting to hold the posture and support the lumbar spine.

Descent: To come out of the pose, the agonists, especially at the hip, must now contract eccentrically (lengthen) to keep the legs from slamming into the floor. In other words, they control the movement toward resistance, or else gravity would cause the downward movement to be too fast.

In *Navasana*, the muscles being stretched are mostly the hamstrings, especially if the knees are straightened. If the arms are forward, the latissimus dorsi, teres major and minor, infraspinatus, posterior deltoid, and triceps are lengthened to some extent. These are muscles located posteriorly (on the back) that extend the shoulder joint. The shoulder girdle is fixed neutrally.

An important note: All muscles have the ability to be agonists, antagonists, synergists, and stabilizers (fixators). The role of the muscle depends on the movement being performed. A muscle can be a primary mover, and other muscles that can do the same movement are called "synergistic" where they aid the primary muscle or become secondary movers or supporters of the position. Sometimes the term "neutralizer" is used as well as "synergist" when a muscle acts to cancel out an unwanted movement by another muscle (usually a muscle that can work two joints, called "biarticulate"). *Complicated!*

In yoga asanas, it is most important to know which muscles are strengthening (contracting), which muscles are being stretched (lengthened), and which muscles are working as stabilizers to support the pose.

Levers

A lever is a device for transmitting but not creating force and consists of a rigid bar moving about a fixed point (fulcrum). More specifically, a lever consists of an effort force, a resistance force, a rigid bar, and a fulcrum. The bones, joints, and muscles together form a system of levers in the body, where the joints act as fulcrums, the muscles apply the effort, and the bones carry the weight of the body parts to be moved. Levers are classified according to the position of the fulcrum, resistance (load), and effort relative to each other.

In a first-class lever, the effort and resistance are located on opposite sides of the fulcrum. In a second-class lever, the effort and resistance are located on the same side of the fulcrum, and the resistance is between the fulcrum and the effort. Finally, in a third-class lever, the effort and resistance are located on the same side of the fulcrum, but the effort acts between the fulcrum and the resistance; this is the most common type of lever in the human body.

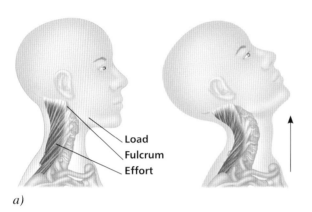

a)

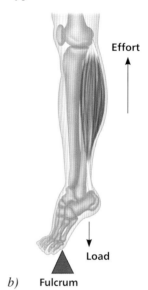

b)

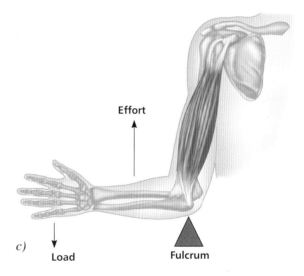

c)

Figure 1.45: Examples of levers in the human body: a) First-class lever; b) Second-class lever; c) Third-class lever.

2 Muscles of Respiration

Yoga and Breath

Breathing is the essence of yoga and one of the main reasons the practice is so vital (notice the first "awareness" of every asana pictured: Breath). Yoga consciously connects the mind and body through attention to breath work, unifying the body processes as the breath heals, nourishes, cleanses, and energizes. Called *prana*, the breath is the awakened life force, as compared to *kundalini*, the dormant energy. Yoga invests prana to discover the latent energy.

In Sanskrit (yoga's language) breath work is *pranayama*, the fourth of eight limbs described in the ancient yoga sutras of Patanjali. Different techniques are used to influence the flow, rate, and volume of air through the respiratory system in a conscious way, enabling one to link the mind/body to the unconscious. Examples are *Ujjayi* (Ocean Breath) and *Nadi Shodhana* (Alternate Nostril Breath).

During asanas, the breath becomes regulated with movement: the inhalation is used to expand and the exhalation to release. The forces of prana and apana are apparent here: *prana* is taking breath in for nourishment and healing, and *apana* ("that which takes away") is the down/out action of elimination.[3]

Focus on breath is also used in relaxation methods to quiet the active mind.

In *The Vital Psoas Muscle* (Staugaard-Jones 2012) I stated that the psoas major and the diaphragm, the main breathing muscle, come together at a point known as the "solar plexus." This is an area around the navel and upper lumbar spine that houses a central nerve complex. Within the subtle energy system known as the "chakras," *Manipura*, the third chakra, exists at this junction, where breath is a vital component. Physical, emotional, and spiritual aspects deeply connect here. Chakras will be discussed in more detail in Chapter 5.

The Act of Breathing

Respiration is the process of inhalation and exhalation, stimulating the flow of air, fluids, nerve conduction, and energetic force down to the cellular level. The mechanism is multifaceted and happens naturally.

The dome-shaped diaphragm muscle rhythmically contracts and relaxes to change pressure and volume in the thoracic cavity through the ANS, which controls involuntary actions. As one takes air in, the diaphragm contracts to allow the rib cage and lungs to expand. The diaphragm gets its signal from the phrenic nerve, causing sensation in the diaphragm's central tendon. This area is drawn in by contraction as one inhales, which enables the thoracic cavity to increase in volume and decrease in pressure. Upon exhalation, this is reversed: the capacity is decreased and the pressure is increased, much like a balloon expelling air.

The abdominal cavity is also active. The shape of the belly and spine can change as the diaphragm pushes the belly down and out on inhalation and allows the abdominals to fall back on exhalation. In yoga this is called "belly breath," and is accomplished when the attachments of the muscle on the rib cage, sternum, and lumbar spine are fixed. "Chest breathing" is associated with the central tendon (top portion) of the diaphragm being fixed. Other muscles also aid in stabilization and accompany diaphragmatic action.

---

3   *Prana* and *apana* are two of the five *vayus* (*vayu* = Lord of the Winds) that are used in yoga to govern breath work through different body areas in various ways. The other three are *samana* (balanced breath centered around the navel), *udana* (upward movement around the throat), and *vyana* (whole body circulation and expansiveness).

DIAPHRAGM

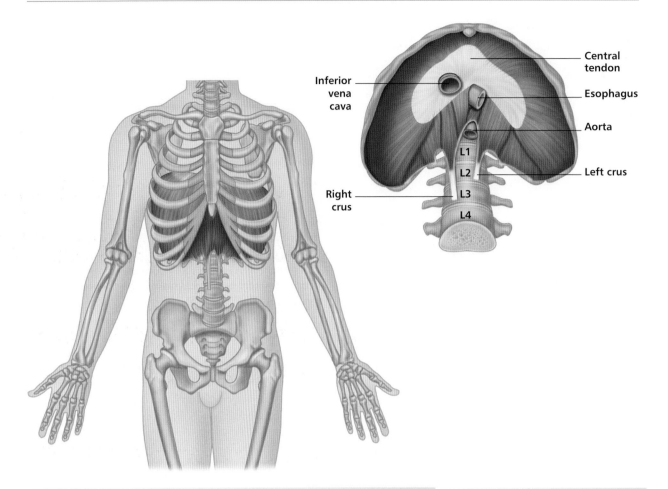

Inferior
vena
cava

Right
crus

Central
tendon

Esophagus

Aorta

Left crus

L1
L2
L3
L4

Greek, *dia*, across; *phragma*, partition, wall.

Origin
Sternal portion: Back of xiphoid process.
Costal portion: Inner surfaces of lower six ribs and their costal cartilages.
Lumbar portion: Upper two or three lumbar vertebrae (L1–L3). Medial and lateral lumbocostal arches (also known as the "medial and lateral arcuate ligaments").

Insertion
All fibers converge and attach onto a central tendon, i.e., this muscle inserts upon itself.

Action
Forms floor of thoracic cavity. Pulls its central tendon downward during inhalation, thereby increasing volume of thoracic cavity.

Nerve
Phrenic nerve (ventral rami), C3, C4, C5.

Functional movement
Produces about 60% of breathing capacity.

Asanas that heavily use this muscle
All asanas, as well as pranayamas.

The diaphragm is pictured in *Vajrasana* (Kneeling Pose) under "Scaleni."

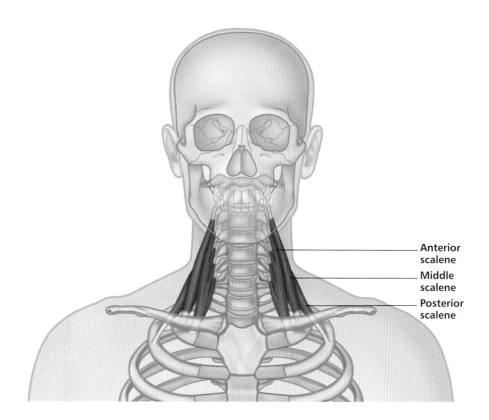

Anterior scalene
Middle scalene
Posterior scalene

Along with the intercostals, the scaleni form part of the accessory muscles of inspiration.

Greek, *skalenos*, uneven. **Latin**, *anterior*, in front; *medius*, middle; *posterior*, behind.

Origin
Transverse processes of cervical vertebrae.

Insertion
Anterior and medius: First rib. Posterior: Second rib.

Action
Acting together: Flex neck. Raise first rib during a strong inhalation. Individually: Laterally flex and rotate neck.

Nerve
Ventral rami of cervical nerves, C3–C8.

Functional movement
The scaleni are primarily muscles of inspiration.

Common problems when muscles are chronically tight or shortened
Painful conditions of the neck, shoulder, and arm, because hypertonic muscle puts pressure on a bundle of nerves called the "brachial plexus" and on the subclavian artery.

Asanas/movements that heavily use these muscles
Strengthening: *Vajrasana* (Kneeling Pose), lifting rib cage during inhale. *Apanasana* (Wind Reliever). Pranayamas.
Stretching: Cervical Circles. Any downward movement of rib cage on exhale.

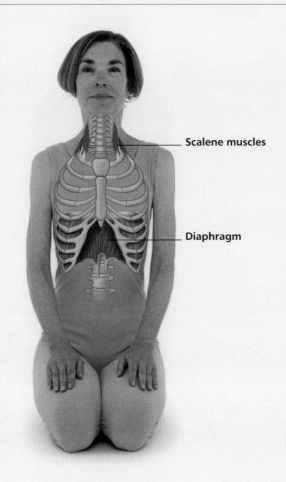

Scalene muscles

Diaphragm

vajra = diamond, thunderbolt; (vaj-RAHS-anna)

Awareness: Breath, rib cage expansion, centering, chakras.

Action and Alignment: Spine extension, shoulder and girdle neutral, hip and knee flexion. Weight of the torso is directly above the sit bones. Viewed from the side, the mid-ear, shoulder, and hip are aligned with each other.

Technique: Begin kneeling with the sit bones on the heels (toes can be tucked under or extended). The spine is lengthened. This can be performed at any time when the practitioner needs to focus inward.

Helpful Hints: This posture is ideal for many pranayamas and/ or meditation. If sitting upright with the legs underneath is uncomfortable, a block or blanket may be used under the sit bones or between the thighs and calves, as raising the hips will accommodate the knees to an easier bend, and put less stress on the ankles and feet. It is recommended to hold this position no longer than ten minutes.

Counter Pose: *Purvottanasana* (see Chapter 6).

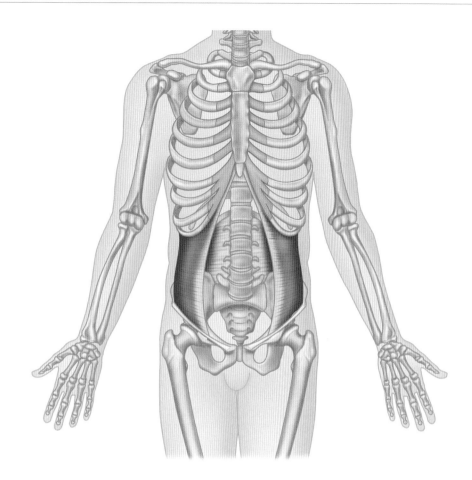

The transversus abdominis is one of the accessory muscles of expiration.

Latin, *transversus*, across; *abdominis*, of the belly/stomach.

Origin
Anterior two-thirds of iliac crest. Lateral third of inguinal ligament. Costal cartilages of lower six ribs. Thoracolumbar fascia.

Insertion
Linea alba via abdominal aponeurosis (tendinous band extending between the sternum and pubis).

Action
Compresses abdomen, helping to support the abdominal viscera against the pull of gravity.

Nerve
Ventral rami of thoracic nerves T7–T12, ilioinguinal and iliohypogastric nerves.

Functional movement
Important during forced expiration, sneezing, and coughing. Helps maintain good posture.

Common problems when muscle is weak
Injury to lumbar spine, because abdominal muscle tone contributes to stability of lumbar spine.

Asanas that heavily use this muscle
Strengthening: Any asana where a forced exhale can be incorporated, such as *Agni Sara* (Fire Cascade). *Bidalasana* (Cat). *Adho Mukha Svanasana* (Down Dog). *Uttihiti Chaturanga Dandasana* (Plank).
Stretching: *Bitilasana* (Cow). *Setu Bhandasana* (Bridge). Strong inhalation.

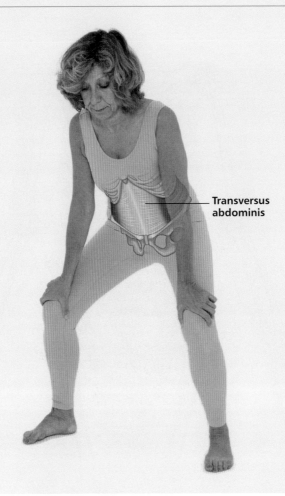

Transversus abdominis

agni = fire; *sara* = essence, waterfall; (AHG-ni Sar-ah) Note: *Agni Sara* is not a posture in the true sense of the word, but more a dynamic practice.

Awareness: Breath, solar plexus, power, pelvic floor (perineum) and rectal lift, abdominal squeeze.

Action and Alignment: Spinal flexion and extension, shoulder and girdle neutral, elbow extension, pelvic tilt, slight hip and knee flexion. Knees are in line with toes, spine is neutral at beginning, shoulders are down.

Technique: Standing with feet at least shoulder-width apart, bend knees and support torso by placing the hands above the knees. The abdominals are activated by expanding on the inhale (spine extension) and contracting inward on the exhale (spine flexion). Repeat three to five times. The transversus abdominis is engaged with a forceful exhale, bringing the belly toward the spine in deep flexion. The "fire" is created in the solar plexus, the third chakra, *Manipura* (see "Chakras" in Chapter 5).

Helpful Hints: This is a powerful, active posture that heats up the central core and affects the interior of the body. Do more gently if pregnant or menstruating, or if there is a hiatal hernia or there are cardiovascular issues. This asana can be performed at any time during the practice, but seems most effective at the beginning or midway point, when warmth is needed.

Counter Pose: *Tadasana* (see Chapter 3).

INTERCOSTALES EXTERNI (External Intercostals)

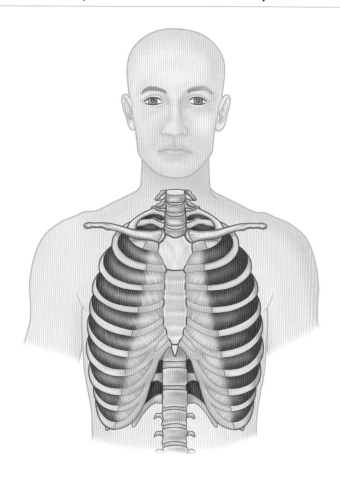

Along with the scaleni and intercostales interni, the intercostales externi are part of the accessory muscles of inspiration.

Latin, *inter*, between; *costa*, rib; *externi*, external.

The lower external intercostal muscles may blend with the fibers of the external oblique, which overlap them, thus effectively forming one continuous sheet of muscle, with the external intercostal fibers seemingly stranded between the ribs. There are eleven external intercostals on each side of the rib cage.

Origin
Lower border of a rib.

Insertion
Upper border of rib below (fibers run obliquely forward and downward).

Action
Muscles contract to stabilize the rib cage during various movements of the trunk.
May elevate ribs during inspiration, thus increasing volume of thoracic cavity (although this action is disputed).
Prevents the intercostal space from bulging out or sucking in during respiration.

Nerve
The corresponding intercostal nerves.

Asanas that heavily use the intercostals
Strengthening/Stabilizing:
Virabhadrasana I, II, III (Warriors). *Trikonasana* (Triangle). *Sirsasana* (Headstand). *Vasisthasana* (Side Plank) and High Plank. *Adho Mukha Vrksasana* (Handstand).
Stretching: *Matsyasana* (Fish Pose). Strong inhalation, pranayamas.

INTERCOSTALES INTERNI (Internal Intercostals)

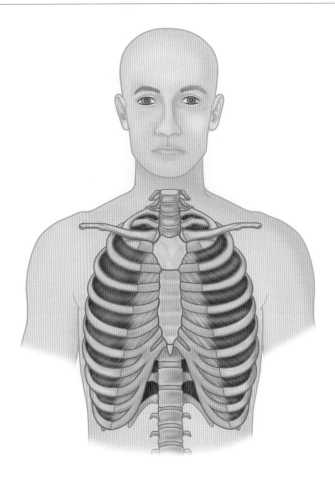

Along with the scaleni and intercostales externi, the intercostales interni are part of the accessory muscles of inspiration.

Latin, *inter*, between; *costa*, rib; *interni*, internal.

Internal intercostal fibers lie deep to and run obliquely across the external intercostals. There are eleven internal intercostals on each side of the rib cage.

Origin
Upper border of a rib and costal cartilage.

Insertion
Lower border of rib above (fibers run obliquely forward and upward toward the costal cartilage).

Action
Muscles contract to stabilize the rib cage during various movements of the trunk.

May draw adjacent ribs together during forced expiration, thus decreasing volume of thoracic cavity (although this action is disputed).

Prevents the intercostal space from bulging out or sucking in during respiration.

Nerve
Corresponding intercostal nerves.

Asanas that heavily use the intercostals
Strengthening/Stabilizing:
Virabhadrasana I, II, III (Warriors). *Trikonasana* (Triangle). *Sirsasana* (Headstand). *Vasisthasana* (Side Plank) and High Plank. *Adho Mukha Vrksasana* (Handstand).
Stretching: *Matsyasana* (Fish Pose). Strong inhalation, pranayamas.

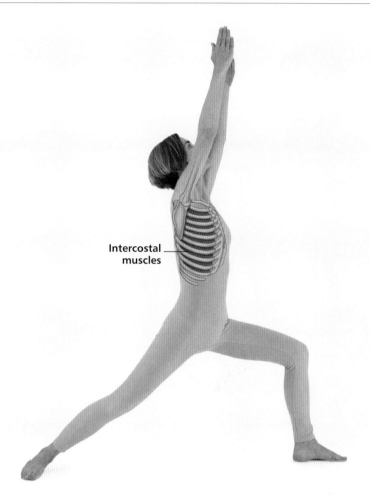

Intercostal muscles

Virabhadra = warrior or super-being from Indian mythology; (veer-ah-bah-DRAHS-anna)

Awareness: Breath, strength, stretch, rib cage expansion, core engagement, *drishti* (focus).

Action and Alignment: Spine extension to hyperextension, shoulder flexion, shoulder girdle elevation to depression, hip and knee flexion (front leg), hip and knee extension (back leg). Pelvis square to the front, front knee directly over ankle, back foot no more than a 45-degree angle from front, front heel in line with middle of back foot arch.

Technique: Stand in *Tadasana*, hands on hips; step back with one leg and position the lower body as stated above, bending the front knee. Inhale and lift arms as demonstrated, eyes forward or up. Two variations can be performed: one with the back foot

at 45 degrees (only if the hips can still be squared to the front), and one with the back foot forward to aid in squaring the pelvis to the front (the stance would be more narrow). The core engages by dropping the tailbone, lifting the pelvic floor, and pulling the abdominals in and up.

Helpful Hints: This is a vigorous posture that helps warm up the body, if done toward the beginning of class, and is also used as a transitional pose. Focus on the breath and soften the intensity. Engage the core to protect the lower spine. Make sure the front knee is facing forward and not hiding the big toe. Press the outside edge of the back foot into the ground and pull energy from the ground up. Both feet are the foundation.

Counter Pose: *Tadasana* (see Chapter 3, add Side Bends).

GLOTTIS AND UJJAYI

Ujjayi (Ocean Breath) is a three-part breath that takes air into the belly, then the mid-chest, and up through the upper chest; the process is reversed on exhalation. An ocean sound is created through the nostrils and resonates in the throat, as the glottis (the space between the vocal folds) is controlled by the larynx muscles to increase or decrease the area according to need. Sounds emanate from this space, as in voice pronunciation. When tension in the folds is changed, the ocean sound can be produced. *Ujjayi* is a warming and very grounding breath used in pranayamas and asanas.

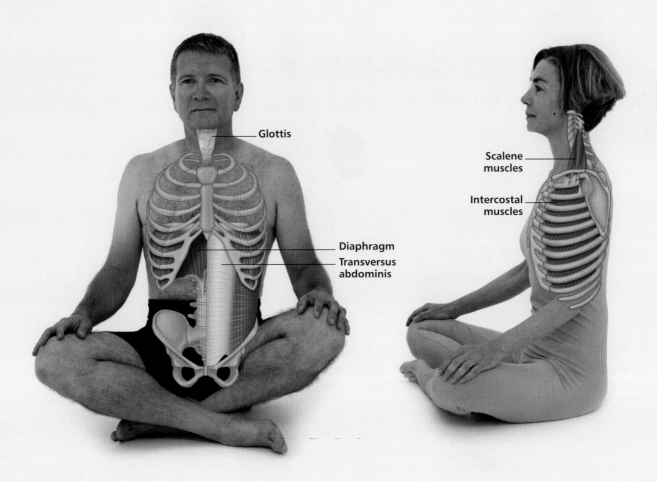

Glottis

Scalene muscles

Intercostal muscles

Diaphragm

Transversus abdominis

sukha = easy, comfortable, happy; (suk-HAS-anna)

Awareness: Breath, ease, centering.

Action and Alignment: Spinal extension, shoulder and girdle neutral, hip flexion and outward rotation, knee flexion. Weight of the torso is directly above the sit bones, with equal weight on both.

Technique: Cross the legs in a sitting position. Lengthen the spine and rest the hands on the thighs, in the lap, or extended on the floor.

Helpful Hints: This is a wonderful meditation and breathing posture, and can be done at any time during class. It is especially beneficial at the beginning, where balance, centering, and harmony can be introduced. It is best to have the knees lower than the hips to help extend the spine, but for some people this is not "easy." Sitting on a block or blankets will help. Uncross the legs and sit in a chair if there is strain.

Counter Pose: Change the leg that is in front. After the asana has been performed in both leg positions, extend the legs and shake them out.

3

Muscles of the Face, Head, and Neck

Although in today's society yoga is sometimes portrayed as a marketable exercise program, or even as a cult in some circles, the ancient and true goal of yoga is meditation, leading to awareness of the true self, our deepest nature of oneness and infinity. Asanas and pranayamas are practiced to attain this state of unity.

The neck muscles are obviously important for movement of the head, but the muscles of the face and skull must also be included; otherwise, how can one achieve inner peace unless attention is focused on the muscles of concentration, emotion, and tension found in this area? A few of these will be presented here to help the practitioner understand that, as muscles and mechanisms are understood in yoga, a profound knowledge can be gained.

Muscle Relaxation and Contraction: The Motor Unit

The relaxation of certain muscles is paramount if one wishes to achieve correct posturing and release in yoga. Skeletal muscles can be brought under conscious control, as they are linked directly to the somatic nervous system (SNS), which is part of the peripheral nervous system (PNS). The SNS carries information from the nerves to the central nervous system (CNS) and from the CNS to the muscles and sensory fibers; it is associated with voluntary muscle control.

A "motor unit" is defined as the motor neuron (there can be many in a single muscle) and all the muscle fibers it innervates; it is the single connection between the CNS and muscular activity. When the neuron transmits a nerve impulse, the muscle contracts: when the neuron does not transmit an impulse, the muscle relaxes. It has been proven that one has the ability to "train" the motor units to become quiet, allowing relaxation.

In simple terms, a willful decision of the mind can release internal signals to help silence the nerve impulses, resulting in relaxation. Imagine the following face and head muscles at rest, allowing for deeper release of tension. This leads to clarity.

OCCIPITOFRONTALIS

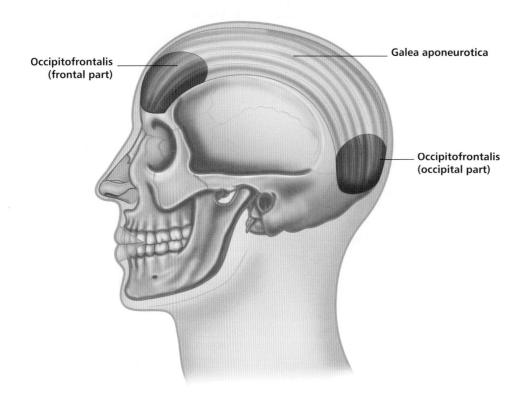

Occipitofrontalis (frontal part)

Galea aponeurotica

Occipitofrontalis (occipital part)

Latin, *occiput*, back of the head; *frontalis*, relating to the front of the head.

This muscle is effectively two muscles (occipitalis and frontalis) united by an aponeurosis called the "galea aponeurotica," so named because it forms what resembles a helmet (Latin *galea*) upon the skull.

Origin
Occipitalis: Occipital bone. Mastoid process of temporal bone. Frontalis: Galea aponeurotica (a sheet-like tendon leading to frontal belly).

Insertion
Occipitalis: Galea aponeurotica. Frontalis: Fascia and skin above eyes and nose.

Action
Occipitalis: Pulls scalp backward. Frontalis: Pulls scalp forward.

Nerve
Facial VII nerve.

Basic functional movement
Example: Raises eyebrows (wrinkles skin of forehead horizontally).

Asanas that heavily use this muscle
Simhasana (Lion Pose).

PLATYSMA

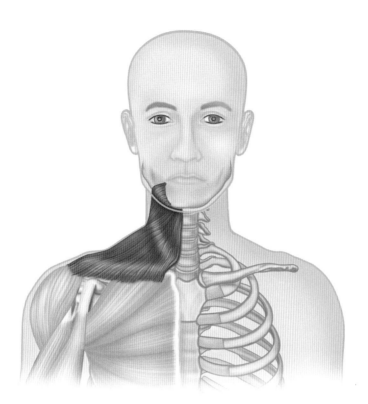

Greek, *platys*, broad, flat.

This muscle may be seen to stand out in a runner finishing a hard race.

Origin
Subcutaneous fascia of upper quarter of chest (fascia overlying pectoralis major and deltoid muscles).

Insertion
Subcutaneous fascia and muscles of chin and jaw. Inferior border of mandible.

Action
Pulls lower lip from corner of mouth downward and laterally. Draws skin of chest upward.

Nerve
Facial VII nerve (cervical branch).

Basic functional movement
Example: Produces expression of being startled or of sudden fright.

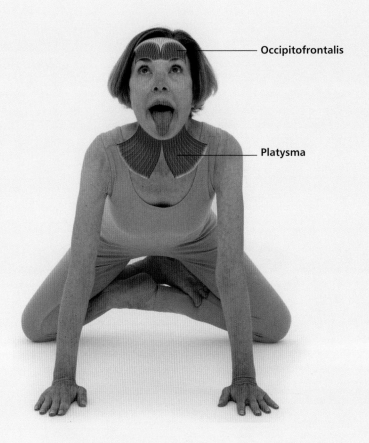

Occipitofrontalis

Platysma

simha = lion; *simhasana* = throne; (sim-HAHS-anna)

Awareness: Breath; release of chest, facial, and breath tension; can engage three major bandhas; benefits chakras 4–6.

Action and Alignment: Spine extension, joints neutral, hip flexion depending on position, facial expression.

Technique: In any sitting meditation position, inhale deeply through the nose, then exhale as the tongue stretches out, curling the tip to the chin. The eyes open wide, with the gaze forward or up toward the eyebrows. A "ha" sound, or sometimes a "roar," is made on the exhale.

Helpful Hints: If body movement is added, one can begin in *Sukhasana* (Easy Pose), then lean onto the hands as the facial expression is performed, bringing the whole torso forward as shown in the illustration. Be mindful of the knees as weight is put upon them in this action. This posture can be added at any point in the class structure.

Counter Pose: Change the front leg if in *Sukhasana*, and then extend and shake out the legs.

NASALIS

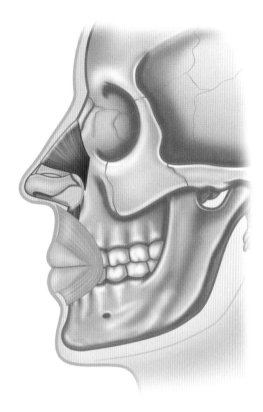

Latin, *nasus*, nose.

Origin
Middle of maxilla (above incisor and canine teeth). Greater alar cartilage. Skin on nose.

Insertion
Joins muscle of opposite side across bridge of nose. Skin at tip of nose.

Action
Maintains opening of external nares during forceful inhalation (i.e., flares the nostrils).

Nerve
Facial VII nerve (buccal branches).

Basic functional movement
Example: Breathing in strongly through the nose.

Pranayamas that heavily use this muscle
Ujjayi (Ocean Breath). *Nadi Shodhana* (Alternate Nostril Breath).

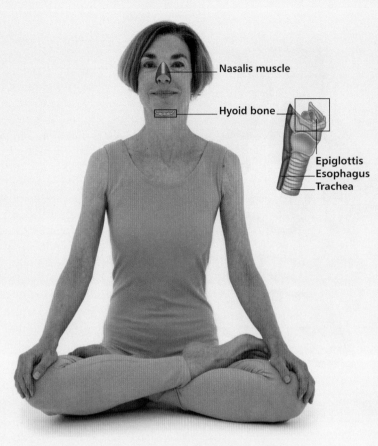

Nasalis muscle

Hyoid bone

Epiglottis
Esophagus
Trachea

A Note About the Hyoid Bone

The hyoid bone is found in the neck area, below the chin and above the larynx. In relation to joints, it is just beneath the jaw. Small and similar to a "wishbone," it surrounds the esophagus. It is an anchoring structure for the tongue and other tissue, but does not articulate with other bones to form a joint. It moves up and down as one swallows and speaks.

The hyoid is mentioned in this text because of placement and the tone of the muscles surrounding that can influence tension and digestion. The tongue is also important in this regard, as it is anchored to the hyoid. It is a connector between muscles in the front and back of the neck. As mentioned in the next section, the sternocleidomastoid (SCM) and spleni muscles (splenius capitis/cervicis) can work in harmony if the hyoid bone is in the right alignment. Think of drawing the top of the throat back and up gently; the back of the neck will extend yet relax along with the front neck muscles, such as the SCM. Smaller, deeper muscles called the "longus capitis/colli" at the front of the cervical spine can then complete their mission: allowing the neck to lengthen even more. Sound like magic? Cueing the suspension of the head in any yoga posture can aid this alignment, releasing tension in connected areas, such as the shoulder girdle and shoulder joints. Reminding the practitioner to extend (but not hyperextend) the neck in backbends might also help in the positioning and conditioning of this entire area.

padma = lotus; (pod-MAHS-anna)

Awareness: The lotus is a symbol of creation, or full bloom; therefore this posture enhances the power of prana.

Action and Alignment: Spine extension, shoulder and girdle neutral, hip flexion and outward rotation, ankle supination, extreme bend of knees and ankles. The mid-ear, shoulder, and hip are aligned.

Technique: Begin in *Sukhasana*, then place one foot into the hip crease of the opposite leg (half Lotus). A full Lotus is completed when both feet are placed into the hip creases without discomfort.

Helpful Hints: A cherished posture of meditation, it can be hard on the hips, knees, and feet. After a half Lotus has been performed, the legs can be changed, for modification. Although it may be done at any time during class, it is especially effective during final contemplation.

Counter Pose: *Dandasana* (see page 49).

TEMPORALIS

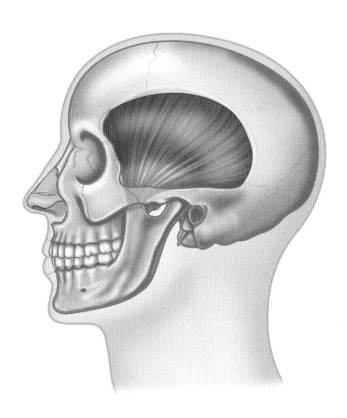

Agonist Versus Antagonist Muscles

Definitions of these muscle functions are given in Chapter 1. Here we will use the following neck muscles to illustrate agonists and antagonists. Opposite in location, as well as in flexion and extension, the sternocleidomastoid (SCM) and spleni muscles, depending on the movement, are each other's agonist and antagonist. For example, in a sit-up or in yoga *Apanasana*, the sternocleidomastoid flexes the neck against gravity (concentric contraction) while the spleni act antagonistically and lengthen. The SCM then contracts eccentrically on the way down, to keep the head from striking the ground.

Usually when the extensors contract concentrically to lift the head (body in a vertical position), the flexors relax. Similarly, when a flexor contracts concentrically, or shortens, the opposing extensor relaxes, even stretching or lengthening, depending on the forces. Remember that agonists are referred to as "the prime movers that contract to perform a specific movement," so their opposite muscles must release to allow this to happen.

Latin, *temporalis*, pertaining to the side of the head.

Origin
Temporal fossa, including parietal, temporal, and frontal bones. Temporal fascia.

Insertion
Coronoid process of mandible. Anterior border of ramus of mandible.

Action
Closes jaw. Clenches teeth. Assists in side-to-side movement of mandible.

Nerve
Anterior and posterior deep temporal nerves from the trigeminal V nerve (mandibular division).

Basic functional movement
Example: Chewing food.

Asanas that heavily use this muscle
Simhasana.

STERNOCLEIDOMASTOIDEUS

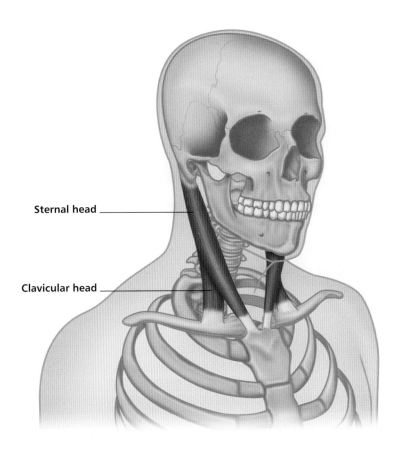

Sternal head

Clavicular head

Greek, *sternon*, chest; *kleis*, key; *mastoeides*, breast shaped.

This muscle is a long strap muscle with two heads. It is sometimes injured at birth and may be partly replaced by fibrous tissue that contracts to produce a torticollis (wry neck).

Origin
Sternal head: Anterior surface of manubrium of sternum.
Clavicular head: Upper surface of medial third of clavicle.

Insertion
Outer surface of mastoid process of temporal bone. Lateral third of superior nuchal line of occipital bone.

Action
Contraction of both sides together: Flexes neck and draws head forward, as in raising the head from a pillow. Raises sternum, and consequently the ribs, superiorly during deep inhalation.
Contraction of one side: Tilts the head toward the same side. Rotates head to face the opposite side (and also upward as it does so).

Nerve
Accessory XI nerve, with sensory supply for proprioception from cervical nerves C2 and C3.

Basic functional movement
Examples: Turning head to look over the shoulder. Raising head from supine position.

Movements or injuries that may damage this muscle
Whiplash, tension.

Common problems when muscle is chronically tight/shortened
Headache, neck pain, inability to hold head up.

Asanas/movement that heavily use this muscle
Strengthening: *Apanasana* (Wind Reliever). *Trikonasana* (Triangle).
Stabilizing: *Dandasana* (Staff Pose).
Stretching: Cervical actions. Looking up, as in *Ustrasana* (Camel), *Matsyasana* (Fish).

Dandasana (Staff Pose) Level I

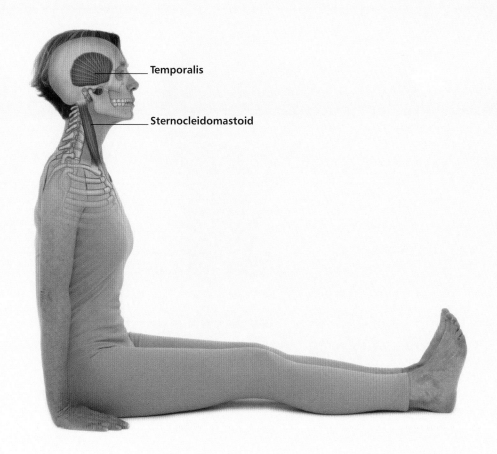

Temporalis

Sternocleidomastoid

danda = staff, rod, stick; (dan-DAHS-anna)

Awareness: Breath, expansion, length, support, core engagement, energetic flow.

Action and Alignment: Spine extension, shoulder and girdle neutral, hip flexion, knee extension, dorsiflexion of ankle. The body makes an "L" shape, with straight spine and legs. Viewed from the side, the ear, shoulder, and hip are in line with each other.

Technique: From any sitting posture, ground with the sit bones and extend the legs out in front. Place the palms of the hands by the sides of the hips on the floor and extend the spine upright as the legs are straightened and held together. Lift the pelvic floor.

Helpful Hints: If there is strain, place a cushion under the knees to soften; some individuals will also benefit by sitting up on a blanket. It is more important to have the spine extended than the knees straightened. Stacking the spine one vertebrae on top of each other is the goal for achieving open energy channels. *Dandasana* can be done at any time during class, especially when the hamstrings need to warm up.

Counter Pose: *Ardha Purvottanasana* (see Chapter 6).

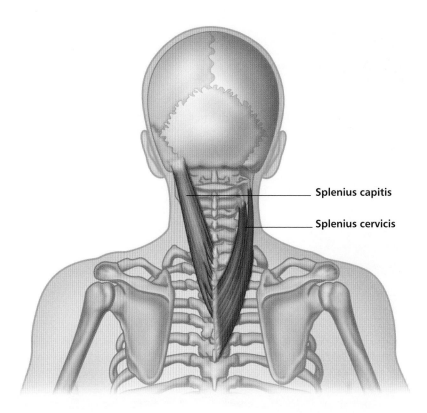

Splenius capitis

Splenius cervicis

Greek, *splenion*, bandage. **Latin**, *capitis*, of the head; *cervicis*, of the neck.

Origin
Splenius capitis: Lower part of ligamentum nuchae. Spinous processes of the seventh cervical vertebra (C7) and upper three or four thoracic vertebrae (T1–T4). Splenius cervicis: Spinous processes of the third to sixth thoracic vertebrae (T3–T6).

Insertion
Splenius capitis: Posterior aspect of mastoid process of temporal bone. Lateral part of superior nuchal line, deep to the attachment of the sternocleidomastoideus. Splenius cervicis: Posterior tubercles of transverse processes of the upper two or three cervical vertebrae (C1–C3).

Action
Acting together: Extend the head and neck.
Individually: Laterally flex the neck. Rotate the face to the same side as the contracting muscle.

Nerve
Dorsal rami of middle and lower cervical nerves.

Basic functional movement
Example: Looking up or turning the head to look behind.

Movements or injuries that may damage this muscle
Whiplash.

Common problems when muscle is chronically tight/shortened
Headache and neck pain.

Asanas/movements that heavily use these muscles
Strengthening: Sitting and standing poses where extension of the neck is important. Forward bends (keeping head in line with spine). Any posture where the head is cued to look up, such as *Virabhadrasana I*.
Stretching: Cervical circles. Chin to Chest.

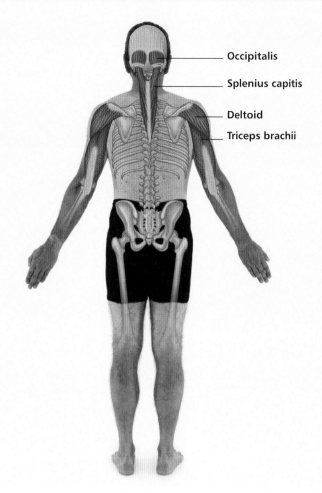

Occipitalis

Splenius capitis

Deltoid

Triceps brachii

tada = mountain; (tah-DAHS-anna)

Awareness: Breath, strength, posture, balance, centering, foundation, inward focus.

Action and Alignment: Spine extension, shoulder neutral, shoulder girdle depression and slight downward rotation, elbow and wrist extension, radioulnar supination, pelvis and hips neutral, knee extension, ankles neutral, toe extension. The mid-ear, shoulder, hip, knee, and anklebone are in alignment with one another.

Technique: Stand with feet parallel and hip-width apart (under anterior hip bones). The feet are the foundation, grounded through the balls of the feet, outside edges, and heels. There is an upward lift in this posture: this affects the arches of the feet, the kneecaps, the pelvic floor and abdominals, and each vertebra up through the top of the head. This is all to create space, energy, and breath.

Helpful Hints: Soften the knees, rib cage, and hyoid bone. Imagine pulling energy up from the earth to the sky while closing the eyes. There is a supported, balanced sensation in this posture, not unlike the peak of a mountain. Try doing this asana against a wall, allowing the shoulder blades, sacrum, and heels to connect to the wall. *Tadasana* is considered the foundation of all standing asanas.

Counter Pose: *Surya Namaskar A* (Salute to the Sun)—Begin in *Tadasana*; Upward Salute (as shown on the front cover); Swan Dive to *Uttanasana*; Flat back lift forward (*Ardha Uttanasana*), and back to *Uttanasana*; Roll up or come up with flat back (Reverse Swan Dive) to Upward Salute, then to *Tadasana* with hands in prayer position, *Anjali Mudra*.

Tadasana as the foundation pose of all standing asanas makes it most important. Time must be taken to assume the posture, doing a body scan from the feet up to make sure the stance is balanced, aligned, supportive, and energized. All posterior-located muscles could have been pictured here, but most are neutral and acting as stabilizers, not strengtheners. Imagine the seven Chakras in relation to the spine (Chapter 5), and view Tadasana in a Salute position on the front cover to achieve the full effect.

Muscles of the Spine

Spinal Functions

The spine is the center of the body's universe, from a mechanical point of view as well as an energetic one, since the main chakras also exist here. The spine is active in all asanas, even in a restful state like *Savasana*, where it acts as a conduit for subtle energies and messaging. The spine supports and balances the trunk and head in standing, sitting, kneeling, backbending, and arm-balance postures. It connects the upper and lower extremities and protects the spinal cord, which merges with the brain. Along with the articulating ribs, the thoracic spine houses the heart and lungs, and the lumbar/sacral areas protect sexual and other organs.

The muscles that work the spine stabilize and move its four different areas: cervical, thoracic, lumbar, and sacral (minimal movement here). The fifth section, the coccyx, is immovable because its vertebrae are fused, but it does provide support and protection as weight is transferred while sitting. Thought of as the remnants of a tail in the evolutionary process, the coccyx maintains another purpose in the human body—that of attachment points of muscles and ligaments, mostly of the pelvic floor.

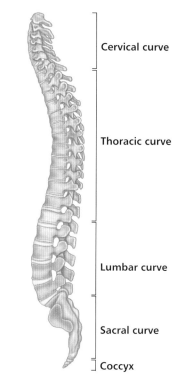

Cervical curve

Thoracic curve

Lumbar curve

Sacral curve

Coccyx

Spine, lateral view.

Spinal Actions

The top three mobile areas of the spine can do the actions of flexion, extension, lateral flexion to the right and left, and rotation to the right and left. The spine is also capable of hyperextension (backbending). There are, however, some limitations of spinal movements.

Cervical—Considered the most movable area of the spine as it curves anteriorly (lordotic) to balance the weight of the head, the top two vertebral joints are limited in some joint actions. The atlanto-occipital joint (between the skull and the C1 vertebra, called the "atlas") can flex and extend (nodding the head), with very little lateral flexion and no rotation. The atlanto-axial joint (between C1, atlas, and C2, axis) mostly rotates. All other cervical vertebral joints (C3–C7) are able to move freely in all three planes if there are no complications.

As in any yoga posture, a main goal is to create space in the body, not condense it; that is why I instruct a student to extend, not hyperextend, the posterior neck position and to not compress the vertebrae.

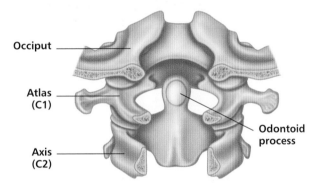

Atlanto-occipital joint.

Thoracic—This is the longest section of the spine, with twelve vertebrae. Its main limitation is hyperextension (arching the back, as in *Ustrasana*, camel pose, see below). The posterior processes of the lower vertebrae in this region begin to slant downward, so when a backbend is performed, one bony process may come in contact with the next. This is very important for yoga practitioners to understand: as the back arches, it cannot be forced into a bone-against-bone position.

Each person is different, but most have a natural kyphotic curve in this section (posterior) and a backbend creates the opposite. *Backbends are aided more by the lordotic areas of the spine (the lumbar and cervical areas), as well as by the upper part*

of the thoracic region, where bony limitation is not as severe. Care and correct explanations must be provided to engage the proper muscles for support of these regions and allow openness of the front of the body.

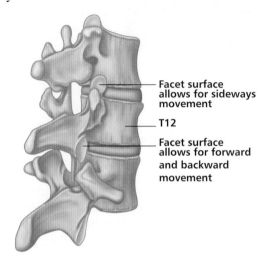

The change in angle between the facet joints lends itself to the movements that are possible at each section of the vertebrae.

Feeling length in the spine as the back bridges will help one perform with more ease and also protect the discs of the spine (cartilage between the vertebrae).

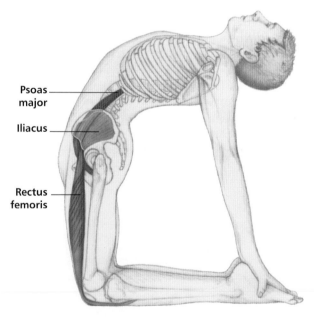

Ustrasana (Camel Pose) Level I-II: anterior muscles pictured are stretching, as posterior muscles located along the spine support the back-bending. Notice the position of the pelvis (in line with the knees) and the cervical area of the spine supporting, not dropping, the weight of the head.

Lumbar—This section of the spine has an anterior curve and contains the five largest and thickest spinal vertebrae. The main limitation is rotation, because of the shape of the bones. The spinal (posterior) processes are bulky, and the facets (articulating surfaces) are orientated in such a way as to limit turning. Once again, this knowledge is of the utmost importance, especially when a spinal twist is performed.

Many injuries of the lower back in yoga can happen because a twist is forced more through the lumbar spine than through the thoracic spine. Overstretching in spinal flexion is also a risk factor.

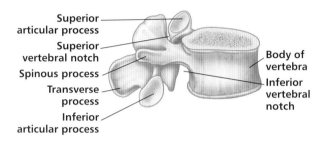

Lumbar vertebra (L3) lateral view.

Sacral—By the end of puberty, four to five vertebrae in this part of the spine have fused together, causing the formation of the sacrum bone, which solidifies through the years and bears the weight of the spinal column. The vertebrae themselves do not move, but at the junction of the sacrum with the pelvis (the sacroiliac, or SI, joint) there is a gliding motion. This is subtle and involuntary; it happens naturally in childbirth as ligaments supporting the joint begin to stretch when the hormone relaxin is released.

Extreme overstretching in yoga (as in Sitting Forward Bend, *Paschimottanasana*) can lead to SI joint discomfort, as ligaments cannot easily "bounce back" to their original length. The area becomes less stable, with resulting inflammation and pain. Sitting too much can also irritate this region.

Actions specific to this pelvic area are called "nutation" (forward motion of sacrum base) and "counter-nutation" (backward motion of sacrum base). They should not be confused with pelvic rotation or tilt, although they can happen along with these actions.

In conclusion, the sacral area of the spine, although not very movable, can be irritated. This is seen in more advanced yoga postures, and one should take care in intense forward-bending poses, twists, wide-leg straddles, and even backbends.

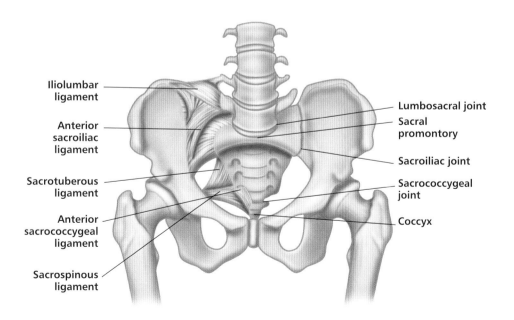

Ligaments around the pelvis and the sacroiliac joint.

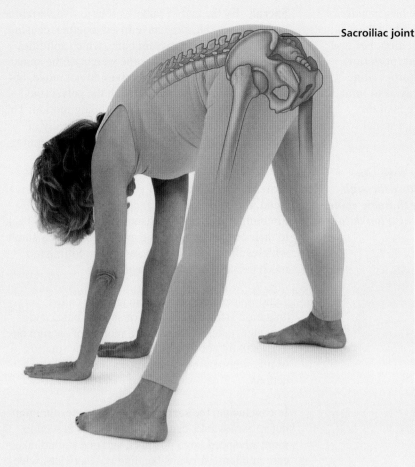

Sacroiliac joint

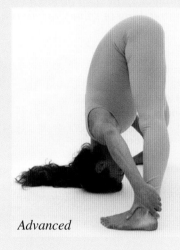

Advanced

prasarita = spread; *pado* = feet; *tan* = expand; (pra-sa-REE-tah pah-doe-tahn-AHS-anna)

Awareness: Breath, expansion, length, stretch, calming, introspection.

Action and Alignment: Spine extension, shoulders and girdle neutral, hip flexion and abduction, knee extension, hamstrings and calf stretch, spreads the SI joint area. Top of the pelvis is brought forward as the hips flex.

Technique: Stand in *Tadasana*, facing the long edge of the mat; open the legs wider than the shoulders, approximately one leg length apart. With hands on hips, inhale and lift the torso, exhale and fold forward from the hips. When the spine is parallel to the floor, take another full breath, extending out and engaging the core. On an exhale, release all the way down, hands coming to a block or the floor. Feel the energy coming from the earth, through the feet and up the legs, engaging the quadriceps to allow the hamstrings to stretch.

Helpful Hints: Once folded forward, there are many variations of this posture, increasing length and space in both the front and the back of the body. Wide-leg Down Dog, spinal twists, and deep lunges can be added for extra benefit. This pose is used to counteract a series of standing asanas.

Counter Pose: *Tadasana* with a slight backbend, hands on sacrum.

Just as the spine is central to the body, so it is to yoga.

The following sections present the major muscles working the spine, with related asanas illustrated and explained in detail.

ERECTOR SPINAE (SACROSPINALIS)

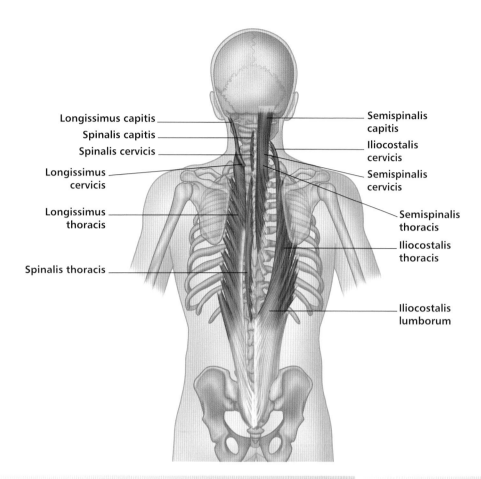

Longissimus capitis
Spinalis capitis
Spinalis cervicis
Longissimus cervicis
Longissimus thoracis
Spinalis thoracis

Semispinalis capitis
Iliocostalis cervicis
Semispinalis cervicis
Semispinalis thoracis
Iliocostalis thoracis
Iliocostalis lumborum

Latin, *erigere*, to erect; *spinae*, of the spine; *sacrum*, sacred; *spinalis*, spinal.

The erector spinae, also called "sacrospinalis," comprises three sets of muscles organized in parallel columns. From lateral to medial, they are the iliocostalis, longissimus, and spinalis.

Origin
Slips of muscle arising from the sacrum. Iliac crest. Spinous and transverse processes of vertebrae. Ribs.

Insertion
Ribs. Transverse and spinous processes of vertebrae. Occipital bone.

Action
Extends and laterally flexes vertebral column (i.e., bending backward and sideways). Helps maintain correct curvature of the spine in erect and sitting positions. Steadies the vertebral column on the pelvis during walking.

Nerve
Dorsal rami of cervical, thoracic, and lumbar spinal nerves.

Basic functional movement
Example: Keeps back straight (with correct curvatures), and therefore maintains posture.

Movements that may injure this muscle
Whiplash. Lifting without bending the knees or keeping the back erect. Holding an object too far in front of the body.
In yoga, any hyperextended position that is taken too far for that particular person.
Forward bending to the extreme (as in *Paschimottasana*) may overstretch this muscle.

Common problems when muscle is chronically tight/ shortened
Headache and neck pain.

Asanas that heavily use these muscles
Strengthening: Most sitting and standing postures where the spine is extended in opposition to gravity, such as *Virabhadrasana I, II, III* (Warrior). Backbends, as hyperextension of the spine occurs. *Parighasana, Trikonasana, Utthita Parsvakonasana*, and *Viparita Virabhadrasana* (Reverse Warrior)—all lateral flexion postures. *Tadasana* on return to standing.
Stretching: *Balasana* (Child's Pose), *Halasana* (Plow). Side Bends.

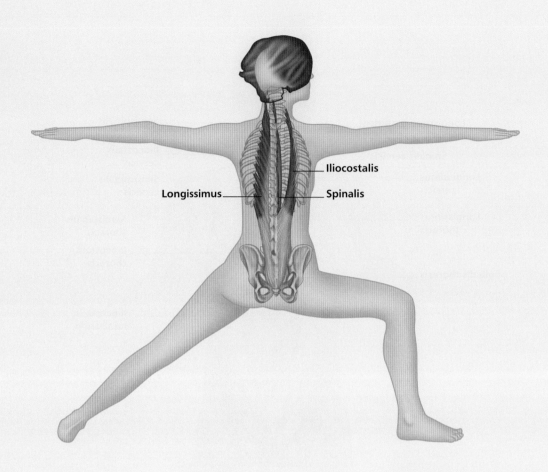

Iliocostalis

Longissimus

Spinalis

Virabhadra = warrior or super-being from Indian mythology; (veer-ah-bah-DRAHS-anna)

Awareness: Breath, space, strength, stretch, rib cage expansion, balance, openness, solidarity.

Action and Alignment: Spine extension, shoulder abduction, shoulder girdle stabilization, hip and knee flexion (front leg), hip extension and abduction, knee extension (back leg). Pelvis open, front knee directly over ankle, back foot at approximately a 90-degree angle from front, front heel in line with middle of back foot arch.

Technique: Stand in *Tadasana*, hands on hips; step back with one leg and position the lower body as stated above, bending the front knee. Inhale and extend the arms out to the sides, eyes forward over the front arm with a strong focus. Engage the core and lift the pelvic floor.

Helpful Hints: A powerful posture that balances the body, it can be done during the beginning to middle of class. This asana can also transition from or to others, such as Warrior I and Triangle. Focus on breath, energy, and extension of the body. Allow the tailbone to drop as the belly lifts; this will protect the lower spine. Make sure the front knee is facing forward and not hiding the big toe, creating slight outward rotation of the front hip. Press the outside edge of the back foot into the ground and pull energy from the ground up. The feet are the foundation.

Counter Pose: Switch sides, then *Tadasana* or *Prasarita Padottanasana* to counter.

SEMISPINALIS CAPITIS, CERVICIS, THORACIS

Transversospinalis (meaning "across the spine") is a composite of three small muscle groups situated deep to erector spinae. However, unlike erector spinae, each group lies successively deeper below the surface, rather than side by side. From the most superficial to the deepest, the muscle groups are semispinalis, multifidus, and rotatores. Their fibers generally extend upward and medially from the transverse processes to the higher spinous processes and are sometimes grouped as the "deep posterior muscles." The combined actions are mostly rotation and extension, with some lateral flexion.

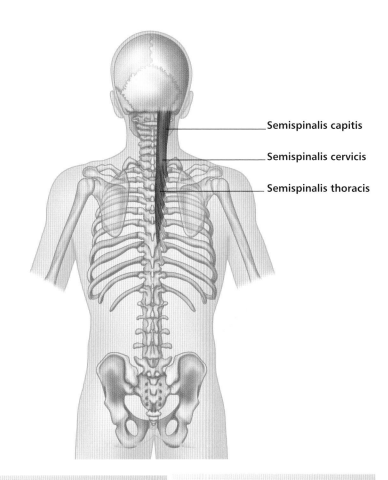

Semispinalis capitis

Semispinalis cervicis

Semispinalis thoracis

Latin, *semispinalis*, half-spinal; *capitis*, of the head; *cervicis*, of the neck; *thoracis*, of the chest.

Origin
Transverse processes of cervical and thoracic vertebrae (C1–T10).

Insertion
Between nuchal lines of occipital bone and spinous processes of the cervical vertebrae and upper four thoracic vertebrae (C2–T4).

Action
Capitis: Most powerful extensor of the head and assists in rotation. Cervicis and thoracis: Extend cervical and thoracic parts of vertebral column. Assist rotation of cervical and thoracic vertebrae.

Nerve
Dorsal rami of cervical and thoracic spinal nerves.

Basic functional movement
Example: Looking up or turning the head to look behind.

Movements that may injure this muscle
Whiplash. In yoga, forcing hyperextension and thoracic/cervical rotation.

Asanas that heavily use these muscles
Strengthening: *Bhujangasana* (Cobra Pose). *Salabhasana* (Locust Pose). *Matsyasana* (Fish Pose). All twisting or revolved asanas. *Virabhadrasana III* (Warrior III).
Stretching: *Balasana* (Child's Pose). *Halasana* (Plow). Twists.

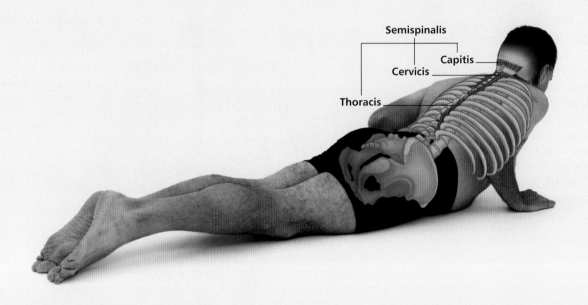

bhujanga = serpent; (boo-jan-GAHS-anna)

Awareness: Breath, strength, stretch, stimulation of core, expansion of heart and lungs (chakra 4).

Action and Alignment: Spine hyperextension, shoulder extension to flexion, shoulder girdle retraction, hip extension. Core and leg engagement, hands directly under the shoulders.

Technique: Lie on the belly, with the hands and elbows into the rib cage. The legs come together and extend, pressing the feet into the floor and engaging the core toward the spine to protect the lumbar area. Lift the torso up from the floor, with the hip bones grounded into the mat. The gaze is forward. The hands are not used to press into the floor; the spinal extensors must contract to lift the upper body against gravity for full benefit.

Helpful Hints: Experience the "baby cobra" first, where the hands can be lifted off the floor to make sure that the spinal extensors are doing the work and not the arms. Once this is established, the hands can then be used to press into the floor and increase the stretch of the front of the body, while the core remains engaged. This is a basic backbend and a good warm-up for more advanced positions; it is included in Sun Salutation to warm up the body. If the lumbar spine is compromised, separate the feet and engage the core more effectively.

Counter Pose: *Balasana* (see Chapter 8).

MULTIFIDUS

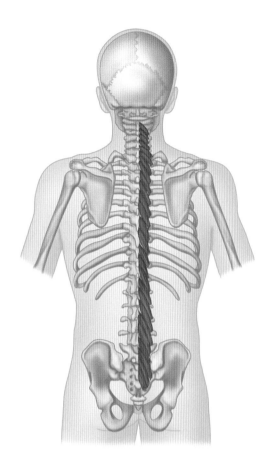

Latin, *multi*, many; *findere*, to split.

This muscle is the part of the transversospinalis group that lies in the furrow between the spines of the vertebrae and their transverse processes.

Origin
Posterior surface of sacrum, between the sacral foramina and posterior superior iliac spine. Mammillary processes (posterior borders of superior articular processes) of all lumbar vertebrae. Transverse processes of all thoracic vertebrae. Articular processes of lower four cervical vertebrae.

Insertion
Parts insert into the spinous process two to four vertebrae superior to the origin; overall, this includes spinous processes of all the vertebrae from the fifth lumbar up to the axis (L5–C2).

Action
Protects vertebral joints from movements made by the more powerful superficial prime movers. Extension, lateral flexion, and rotation of vertebral column.

Nerve
Dorsal rami of spinal nerves.

Basic functional movement
Example: Helps maintain good posture and spinal stability during all movements/asanas.

Movements that may injure this muscle
Lifting without bending the knees or keeping the back erect. Holding an object too far in front of the body when lifting. In yoga, extreme bending or twisting.

Asanas that heavily use this muscle, mainly for stabilization
All standing, kneeling, sitting, backbending, and twisting or revolved asanas.

ROTATORES

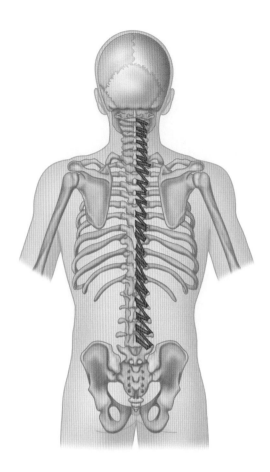

Latin, *rota*, wheel.

These small muscles are the deepest layer of the transversospinalis group.

Origin
Transverse process of each vertebra.

Insertion
Base of the spinous process of adjoining vertebra above.

Action
Rotate and assist in extension of vertebral column.

Nerve
Dorsal rami of spinal nerves.

Basic functional movement
Helps maintain good posture and spinal stability during standing, sitting, and all movements/asanas.

Movements that may injure this muscle
Lifting without bending the knees or keeping the back erect. Holding an object too far in front of the body when lifting. In yoga, twisting the lumbar spine too far is counterproductive.

Asanas that heavily use these muscles
All standing, sitting, and twisting or revolved asanas, both strengthening and stretching

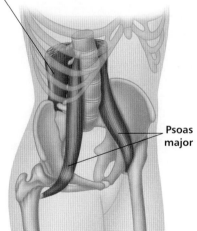

Note the stabilizing effect of the lumbar spine posterior muscles.

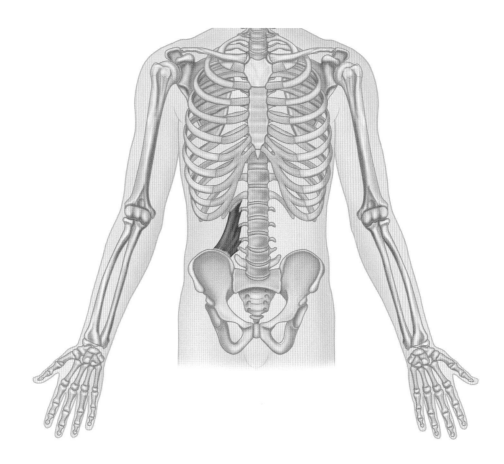

Latin, *quadratus*, four-sided; *lumborum*, of the loins.

A stabilizing muscle.

Origin
Iliac crest. Iliolumbar ligament (the ligament from the fifth lumbar vertebra to the ilium).

Insertion
Twelfth rib. Transverse processes of upper four lumbar vertebrae (L1–L4).

Action
Laterally flexes vertebral column. Fixes the twelfth rib during deep respiration (helps stabilize the diaphragm for singers exercising voice control). Helps extend lumbar part of vertebral column and gives it lateral stability.

Nerve
Ventral rami of the subcostal nerve and upper three or four lumbar nerves (T12, L1, L2, L3).

Basic functional movement
Example: Bending sideways from sitting to pick up an object from the floor.

Movements that may injure this muscle
Bending sideways or lifting from a sideways position too quickly.

Common problems when muscle is chronically tight/shortened
Referred pain to hip and gluteal area, as well as lower back.

Asanas that heavily use this muscle
Strengthening: *Bharadvajasana. Viparita Virabhadrasana. Parighasana. Utthita Parsvakonasana.*
Stretching: *Tadasana* with Side Bend. *Halasana* (Plow).

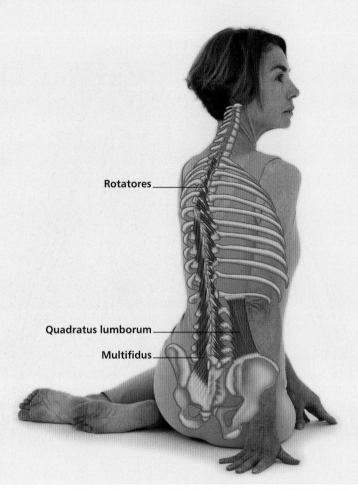

Rotatores

Quadratus lumborum

Multifidus

Bharadvaja = legendary sage; (bah-ROD-va-JAHS-anna)

Awareness: Breath, stretch, cleansing, release.

Action and Alignment: Spinal extension and rotation, shoulder and girdle stabilization, elbow extension, hip and knee flexion. Firm legs, and pelvic and arm support.

Technique: Sit with the legs tucked to one side. Engage the core as the spine lifts and twists away from the knees. With one hand on the outside knee, place the other hand behind and close to the spine on the floor. The gaze can follow the twist, provided it does not compromise the neck.

Helpful Hints: One of the easier twists, *Bharadvajasana* can be done after warming up or before cooling down. The spine can twist best when each vertebra is stacked on top of the other first, before rotation begins. A blanket under either hip can help even the vertebrae as the sit bones anchor toward the floor. The use of a prop under the twisting side may relieve discomfort in the lower back. Variations can be performed with the arms and legs.

Counter Pose: *Baddha Konasana* (see Chapter 8)

EXTERNAL AND INTERNAL OBLIQUES

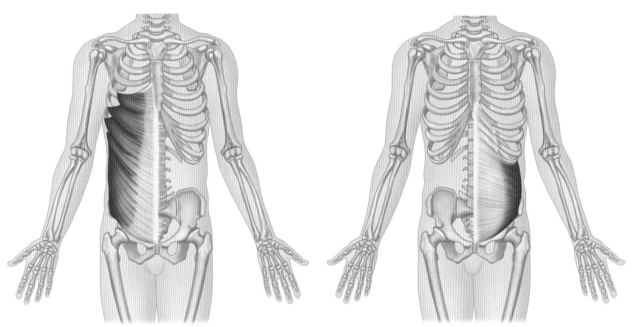

External oblique.

Internal oblique.

Latin, *obliquus*, diagonal, slanted.

The posterior fibers of the external oblique are usually overlapped by the latissimus dorsi, but in some cases there is a space between the two, known as the "lumbar triangle," situated just above the iliac crest. *The lumbar triangle is a weak point in the abdominal wall.* The internal oblique is considered a strong stabilizer as well as a mover.

Origin
External oblique: Lower eight ribs.
Internal oblique: Iliac crest. Lateral two-thirds of inguinal ligament. Thoracolumbar fascia (sheet of connective tissue in lower back).

Insertion
External oblique: Anterior half of iliac crest and into an abdominal aponeurosis that terminates in the linea alba (a tendinous band extending downward from the sternum).
Internal oblique: Bottom three or four ribs and linea alba via an aponeurosis.

Action
Compresses abdomen, helping to support the abdominal viscera against the pull of gravity.
External oblique: Contraction of one side alone bends the trunk laterally and rotates it to the opposite side (contralateral).
Internal oblique: Contraction of one side bends the trunk laterally and rotates it to the same side (ipsilateral).
When right and left sides contract simultaneously (both external and internal obliques) they aid in flexion.

Nerve
External oblique: Ventral rami of thoracic nerves T5–T12.
Internal oblique: Ventral rami of thoracic nerves T7–T12, ilioinguinal and iliohypogastric nerves.

Basic functional movement
Example: Digging with a shovel, raking, twisting.

Common problems when muscles are weak
Injury to lumbar spine, because abdominal muscle tone contributes to stability of lumbar spine.

Asanas that heavily use these muscles
Strengthening: Any asana that laterally bends, flexes, or rotates the spine, such as *Trikonasana, Parighasana, Utthita Parsvakonasana, Ardha Matsyendrasana, Parivrtta Trikonasana. Parivrtta Janu Sirsasana* and *Baddha Parsvakonasana*.
Stretching: Side Bends. *Setu Bhandasana* (Bridge).

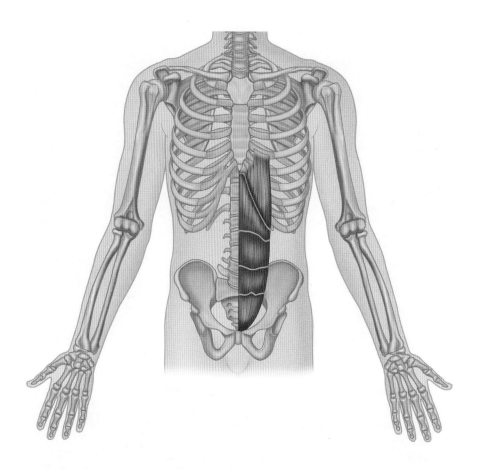

Latin, *rectus*, straight; *abdominis*, of the belly/stomach.

The rectus abdominis is divided into three or four bellies by tendinous bands, each sheathed in aponeurotic fibers from the lateral abdominal muscles. These fibers converge centrally to form the linea alba. Situated anterior to the lower part of the rectus abdominis is a frequently absent muscle called the "pyramidalis," which arises from the pubic crest and inserts into the linea alba. It tenses the linea alba, for reasons unknown. This and the upper rectus abdominis are associated with the six-pack striation seen in conditioned athletes.

Origin
Pubic crest and symphysis (front of pubic bone).

Insertion
Xiphoid process (base of sternum); fifth, sixth, and seventh costal cartilages.

Action
Flexes lumbar spine. Depresses rib cage. Stabilizes the pelvis during walking.

Nerve
Ventral rami of thoracic nerves T5–T12.

Basic functional movement
Example: Initiating getting out of a low chair. Rolling up from a supine position.

Common problems when muscle is weak
Injury to lumbar spine, because abdominal muscle tone contributes to stability of lumbar spine.

Asanas that heavily use this muscle
Strengthening: *Trikonasana. Apanasana. Navasana. Agni Sara. Utkatasana* and others using rectus abdominis as a stabilizer of the spine.
One-leg standing asanas to help stabilize spine and pelvis: *Virabhadrasana III. Vrksasana.*
Stretching: *Setu Bhandasana* (Bridge). Backbends.

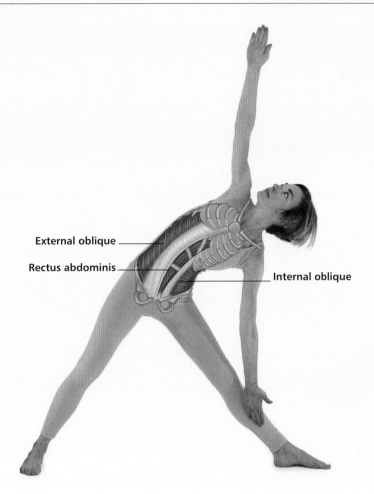

External oblique

Rectus abdominis

Internal oblique

trikona = three angles or triangle; (tree-kone-AHS-anna)

Awareness: Breath, strength, stretch, expansion, balance, support, stimulation, power, therapeutic, centering.

Action and Alignment: Spine extension, shoulder abduction, shoulder girdle stabilization, elbow and wrist extension, core engagement, pelvic stability, hip flexion and outward rotation (front leg), hip extension and abduction (back leg), knee flexion and extension, ankle supination of back foot. Shoulders stacked one over the other, heel of front leg aligned with center of back foot.

Technique: From *Tadasana* with hands on hips, step back with one foot into *Virabhadrasana II*. Extend the front knee without locking, and center the pelvis. Engage the core and lift the pelvic floor. Reach the front arm and torso forward as the pelvis pushes back. Once this position is reached, drop the bottom hand to the inside of the leg or block as the top arm extends to the sky. Keep the head in line with the spine. Hold for up to one minute.

Helpful Hints: The body is extended as if supported between two planes; try the asana with the back of the body against a wall to experience this. Provided the neck is not compromised, the gaze can be up toward the top hand (some practitioners might choose to rest the top hand on the sacrum instead). The hamstrings will be stretched, especially in the back leg; softening the knees will help release the tension. Inhale to lift up and out of the pose, then repeat on the other side. The asana is best when done at the middle of class, where centering is needed.

Counter Pose: *Viparita Virabhadrasana* (see below, under "Psoas Major").

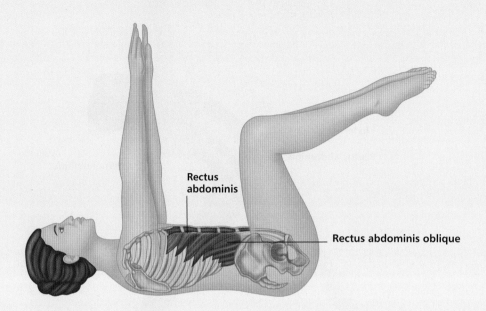

Rectus
abdominis

Rectus abdominis oblique

Another asana that primarily targets the rectus abdominis is *Apanasana* (Wind Reliever). It is similar to the Pilates 100 position. The technique described below will explain the differences.

apa = away; *apana* = one of the five main *vayus* explained in Chapter 2; (ah-pa-NAHS-anna)

Awareness: Breath, core and neck strength, digestion, elimination.

Action and Alignment: Spine flexion, shoulder and girdle stabilization, hip flexion, knee flexion. Knees directly over the hips.

Technique: Lie on the back, with knees bent and shins in Table position. Hands rest on the knees. Inhale, then exhale as the spine flexes and the nose moves toward the knees. Inhale and stretch the legs away, then exhale and bring them back to Table. Inhale and roll down. Repeat three or four times.

Helpful Hints: Use the rectus abdominis to flex the spine, and the SCM to flex the neck. The spine is stretched, as well as the gluteal muscles. This posture is good at the beginning of class, to help warm the core, or at the end, before *Savasana*.

Counter Pose: *Savasana* (see Appendix 1).

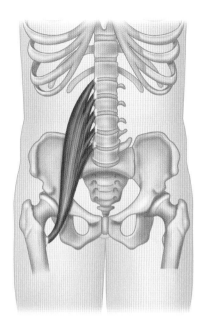

Greek, *psoa*, muscle of the loin.
Latin, *major*, larger.

The psoas major and iliacus (iliopsoas muscle group) are considered part of the posterior abdominal wall because of their position and cushioning role for the abdominal viscera. However, on the basis of their action of flexing the hip joint (the psoas major is the weaker of the two), it would also be relevant to place these two muscles in Chapter 8. The psoas major individually is also a deep core muscle because of its attachment to the lumbar spine (covered in Chapter 5). Note that some of the upper fibers of the psoas major may insert by a long tendon into the iliopubic eminence to form the psoas minor, which has little function and is absent in about 40% of people.

Bilateral contracture of this muscle might increase lumbar lordosis, and overuse or underuse may lead to other postural issues and/or pain—balance is the key!

Origin
Bases of transverse processes of all lumbar vertebrae (L1–L5). Bodies of twelfth thoracic and all lumbar vertebrae (T12–L5). Intervertebral discs above each lumbar vertebra.

Insertion
Lesser trochanter of femur.

Action
Flexor of hip joint, in conjunction with iliacus (flexes and laterally rotates thigh, as in kicking a football). Acting from its Insertion, it weakly flexes the trunk, as in sitting up from a supine position. It is a strong stabilizer at both lumbar spine and hip joints.

Nerve
Ventral rami of lumbar nerves (L1, L2, L3, L4; psoas minor innervated from L1, L2).

Basic functional movement
Example: Going up a step or walking up an incline.

Movements that may injure or compromise this muscle
Overuse, as it is a strong stabilizer, and a biarticulate muscle at the lumbar spine and hip. Underuse, such as sitting too much, which leads to a shortened, atrophied psoas.

Asanas that heavily use this muscle
Any standing asana uses the psoas major as a stabilizer at both lumbar spine and hip joints.
Strengthening: *Navasana. Virabhadrasana I, II, III* (and Reverse Warrior, where strength is in the front leg, and stretch is in the back leg—as pictured). *Alanasana* (lunge, strength is in the front leg).
Stretching: Back leg of *Anjanyasana, Virabhadrasanas, Alanasana.*

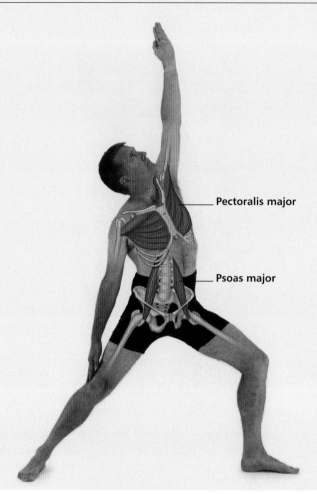

Pectoralis major

Psoas major

viparita = reversed, inverted; *Virabhadra* = name of a warrior; (vip-par-ee-tah veer-ah-bah-DRAHS-anna)

Awareness: Breath, stretch, strength, rib cage expansion, pelvic stability, circulation.

Action and Alignment: Spine lateral flexion, shoulder abduction and adduction, shoulder girdle stabilization, elbow and wrist extension, hip flexion/extension/abduction, knee flexion and extension. Lower body alignment as in Warrior II.

Technique: From *Virabhadrasana II*, reverse the spine and arms up and back, keeping the legs firm and the feet grounded evenly. To increase the challenge, the lunge can be increased and the back arm wrapped behind for a binding effect. Lift the core and pelvic floor as the torso stretches to the back side.

Helpful Hints: A nice counter to Warriors and Triangles, this posture is done more as a side bend than as a backbend. The breath is strong as the body expands on the inhale, and softens in intensity on the exhale.

Counter Pose: *Uttanasana* (see Chapter 6).

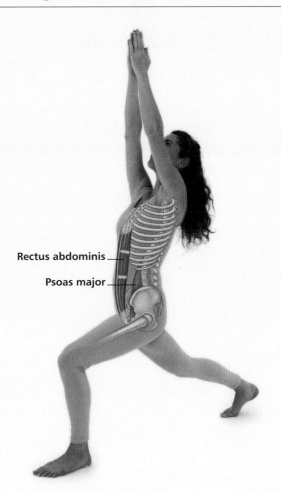

Rectus abdominis

Psoas major

An excellent example of an asana that uses all the muscles discussed in this chapter (as well as the main ones of the hip and knee joints) is *Alanasana* (High Lunge). This asana is especially effective for developing both strength (front leg) and stretch (back leg) for the psoas major, which also acts as a stabilizer for the lumbar spine.

Alana = minister of Shiva; (al-ahn-AHS-anna)

Awareness: Breath, strength, stretch, support, core work, balance, energy, *drishti* (focus).

Action and Alignment: Spine extension, shoulder flexion, shoulder girdle stabilization, hip flexion and extension, knee flexion and extension, core engagement. Front knee is aligned directly above the ankle, with the pelvis centered.

Technique: Usually done during a Sun Salutation before or after a Down Dog. Lift one leg to the back (three-legged Dog), then bring that leg forward with the knee bent, placing the foot between the hands. Lift the torso, either with the hands on the front thigh or with the arms up in the air.

Helpful Hints: Check front knee alignment and engage the core by dropping the tailbone, lifting the lower abdominals and pelvic floor. Energize the back leg by straightening the knee and pushing out through the back heel. A strong gaze forward will be helpful to maintain balance. Blocks may be placed on the outside of both feet for support and balance, as well as resting the back knee on the floor.

Counter Pose: *Adho Mukha Svanasana* (see Chapter 6).

The Deep Core and Pelvic Floor

In Chapter 4 the spine was discussed as the center of the body's universe. The connection of the spine to the pelvis through the sacrum adds the central basin, and the two together become our center of gravity, or core.

The Superficial Versus Deep Core

The surface core is the focus of many exercise programs. The muscles targeted are usually the anterior abdominal muscle group, including three of the four abdominal muscles—the rectus abdominis, and the external and internal obliques. These muscles mostly flex and rotate the thoracic/lumbar spine (Chapter 4).

One must go deeper in order to address the support and health of the entire center of the body. This is where balance, strength, and stability integrate through muscle connection around the lumbar spine. Five hidden yet very important muscles are the diaphragm (lower attachments L1–L3,

page 32), psoas major (page 69), quadratus lumborum (page 63), transversalis group (page 57, minus the semispinalis), and transversus abdominis (page 35, the fourth abdominal muscle). These muscles have already been pictured in the respiration and spine chapters, as they are relevant to and located in these areas. Putting them together helps one see the relationship to the deeper layer of the lower spine and pelvis, the area called the "deep core," where stabilization of the lumbar spine to the pelvis occurs and is necessary for proper alignment of the body.

Asanas That Heavily Use the Deep Core Muscles

All asanas can incorporate the deep core, with special cueing to help the practitioner (see sections on cueing in Appendix 2). Some postures are more useful than others in addressing this area. Starting with breath work will help bring attention to the deep core, and postures of balance and strength can be valuable in discovering the significance of these concealed muscles.

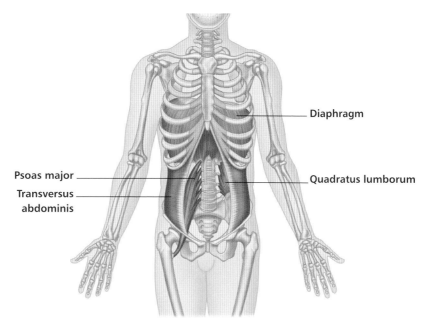

Diaphragm

Quadratus lumborum

Psoas major

Transversus abdominis

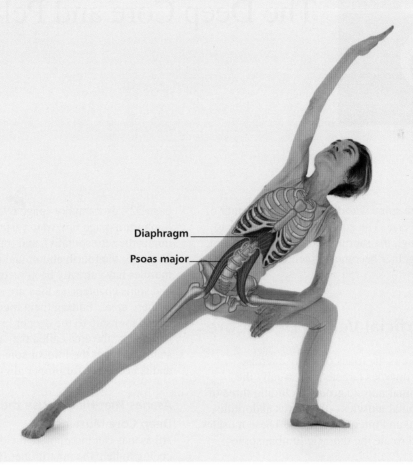

Diaphragm

Psoas major

utthita = extended; *parsva* = sideways; *kona* = angle; (oo-TE-tah parsh-vah-cone-AHS-anna)

Awareness: Breath, strength, stretch, rib cage and chest expansion, core work, balance, centering.

Action and Alignment: Spine extension and lateral flexion, shoulder abduction and adduction, shoulder girdle up-and-down rotation, elbow flexion, hip flexion and extension, knee flexion and extension. A straight angle from the back foot to the top hand is optimal.

Technique: From Warrior II, angle the torso out over the front thigh, support the bottom hand on a block or lightly rest the forearm on the front thigh, and reach the top arm up or alongside the head. The gaze can be down, forward, or up past the high arm. This posture is usually done during a Warrior series, toward the middle of class. The illustration shows the anterior deep core muscles minus the transversus abdominis; imagine how the posterior deep core muscles are also working around the lumbar spine in the role of stabilizers.

Helpful Hints: This is a deep pose where attention is drawn to both legs equally, bringing energy up through the feet and legs, and into the center. Strong cueing for the core is needed here, as well as firm pressure of the back heel into the floor. Relax the neck and shoulders.

Counter Pose: *Viparita Virabhadrasana* (see Chapter 4).

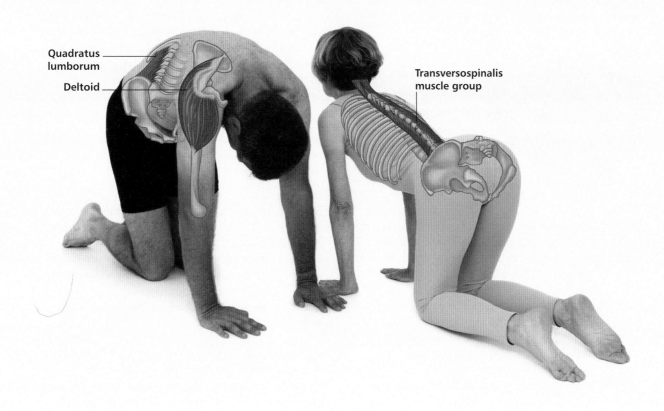

Quadratus lumborum

Deltoid

Transversospinalis muscle group

The Pelvic Floor: Where the Physical Meets the Spiritual

The pelvis is a basin, acting as an architectural keystone to support and balance the two femurs on either side. It is made up of three bones: the sacrum and two iliac bones (fusion of the ilium, ischium, and pubis areas to create the iliac bones happens by or during puberty).

The pelvis can move through space, but the action really occurs at the lumbar spine and iliofemoral (hip) joints, such as in pelvic tilting. Cat and Dog/Cow positions incorporate forward and backward tilt of the pelvis and can be a part of other asanas when cued.

chakra = wheel; *vaka* =crane, mythical bird; (chak-rah-vah-KAHS-anna)
(Separately: *bidalasana* = cat; *bitilasana* = cow)

Awareness: Breath, stretch, strength, pelvic tilt, balance, fluid movement, flexible spine, core, chakras.

Action and Alignment: Spine flexion (cat), spine hyperextension (cow), shoulder flexion, shoulder girdle abduction and adduction, elbow and wrist extension, arm and leg support. Hands are under the shoulders, and knees under the hips.

Technique: From a Table position (prone on hands and knees) begin with the spine in its own neutral curvature. Deepen the anterior curve on the inhale, lifting the tailbone and head as the belly drops (cow back/dog tilt). Exhale as the tailbone drops, rounding the

spine up to a posterior curve; the head drops and shoulder blades separate. Be conscious of how the front of the torso is moving, as well as the back of the body.

Helpful Hints: Initiate all movement from the tailbone, allowing the movement to flow up through the spine. The Sunbird is the balancing portion: from Table, release one arm forward and the opposite leg back. Engaging the core will strongly aid the balance. This is an ideal pose to aid back pain. Hands can be placed on a chair if the arms cannot support the body well. A blanket under the knees might also be helpful. This posture can be done at any time in class, and is especially beneficial for warming up the spine and core.

Counter Pose: *Balasana* (see Chapter 8).

The bottom of this area, the pelvic floor, is unique and especially important in yoga. The many facets and structures are worth investigating, as they enhance breath, posture, balance, and vitality.

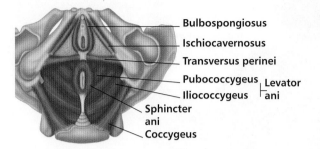

- Bulbospongiosus
- Ischiocavernosus
- Transversus perinei
- Pubococcygeus ⎤ Levator
- Iliococcygeus ⎦ ani
- Sphincter ani
- Coccygeus

Understanding this area and its use is complicated but necessary in most yoga practices. There is another diaphragm here, the pelvic diaphragm, which includes layers of muscle and fascia, as well as the sacral nerve plexus. It is somewhat coordinated with yet a third diaphragm located in the throat, the vocal diaphragm, when breathing. Suffice it to say the pelvic area is most interesting to yogis because of muscular support, sensitive nerve endings, and breath work.

In yoga, we "lift" the pelvic floor. This is a bit ambiguous, but the image of pulling up the bottom of the pelvis aids in engaging the correct musculature, whether in sitting, kneeling, standing, and even inverted postures. This action increases support, balance, and strength of particularly small but necessary muscles. These muscles include the levator ani and coccygeus and other muscles that, when engaged, can strengthen the pelvic floor. The lower abdominal wall is also involved, as well as the psoas major, as a stabilizer. Even the hip adductors can be targeted to help lift the pelvic floor.

The perineum is an area between the inner thighs, in between the urethra and the anus, with the pelvic diaphragm as its roof. It all forms a diamond shape, with two triangles intersected by an imaginary line between the sit bones—the urogenital and anal triangles. Sphincter muscles (ani and urethral) are located here (sphincters are circular muscles that control the flow of material). This is also the location of the engagement of the first *bandha*, or lock, which is meant to raise subtle energy fields to a higher level (see "Bandhas" section below).

When practicing or teaching yoga, a distinction must be made between engaging the pelvic floor and activating the bandhas. When using the pelvic floor to support postures, there is a small, intentional contraction of muscles to lift upward. To activate the bandhas, controlled breathing, along with contraction done in a binding (or held) fashion, is ultimately performed to attain detachment from external senses and release energy up through the spine.

Yoga Philosophy: Bandhas, Nadis, Chakras, and Limbs

Bandhas

There are four major bandhas incorporated in yogic styles: *mula bandha* (perineum and anus), *uddiyana bandha* (abdomen), *jalandhara bandha* (throat), and *jivha bandha* (tongue and palate). Breath work incorporated into Kundalini Yoga is a good example of using all four when appropriately cued. The two lower ones are discussed here, as they relate to the pelvic area.

Mula bandha is the lock associated with the pelvic floor, specifically the perineum and anus. This is a neuromuscular junction that is stimulated by focused concentration and contraction of the area (similar action is present in all four bandhas). This is voluntary and deliberate, where a sensation can be felt as energy is tapped, and a contraction is held to engage an impulse that would release upward through the spine.

Uddiyana bandha is a good example of "flying upward," the literal definition of the Sanskrit term. The low, mid-abdomen, diaphragm, and ribs are focused areas where there is an ascending movement of the diaphragm while the abdominals are concave. It is mentioned here because of the interaction of the pelvic floor muscles with both *mula bandha* and *uddiyana bandha*. Study of these is best done with a master, with the most important aim being a progressive feeling arising out of sustained contraction and not thinking about what is being activated muscularly.

Bandha work becomes part of a sustained practice of yoga asanas and pranayamas. Its goal is the higher aspects of the spiritual path, where the chakras and nadis are important. Awareness becomes internal more than external, allowing for deeper meditation, where enlightenment, known as *Samadhi* (the eighth limb of yoga), can become a possibility.

Upavesasana (Sitting-down Pose) or *Malasana* (Garland Pose) Level I, II

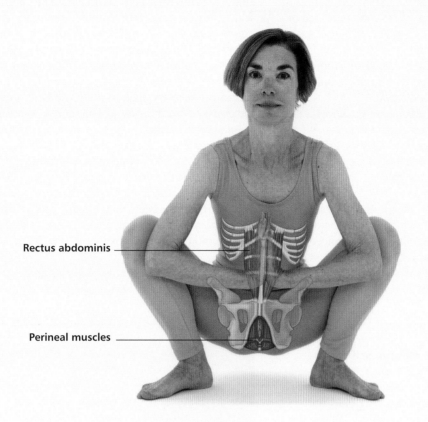

Rectus abdominis

Perineal muscles

upa = toward, down; *maalaa* = garland; *mala* = impurities; (oo-pah-veh-SAHS-anna; ma-LAHS-anna)

Awareness: Breath, stretch, release, stimulates organs and metabolism, bandha engagement, centering, hip opener.

Action and Alignment: Spine extension, shoulder and girdle stabilization, elbow flexion, wrist and hand extension, hip flexion and outward rotation, knee flexion, ankle dorsiflexion. Feet are wider than shoulders and pointed outward, and hands are in prayer position (*Anjali Mudra*).

Technique: Begin in a standing position, with the feet at least one foot length apart and the hands in prayer position or on the hips. Lower the body down slowly, flexing at the hip and knees as the spine remains as straight as possible. This is a squatting position, with the heels up or down. Use the elbows to press the knees apart for a nice stretch.

Helpful Hints: This is an ideal position for the health of the lower back, allowing gravity to release it. Using a block to sit on will soften the impact on the hips, knees, and ankles. A short Achilles tendon in the back of the heel will necessitate the heels remaining off the floor. Strong bandhas can be created here. It is a good transitional pose from standing to sitting and can be done at any time in class.

Counter Pose: *Savasana* (see Appendix 1).

Nadis

Nadis are channels of energy and motion that can be activated by Kundalini work, or "awakening". As quoted by the Originator of this method in the USA, Yogi Bhajan (October 27th, 1988): "Kundalini Yoga is the science to unite the finite with Infinity, and it's the art to experience Infinity in the finite."

Nadis are also used in the practice of Eastern medicines, such as acupuncture, and in the use of meridians. They connect at the subtle energy points known as the "chakras." Yoga and breath become a means of purifying these channels.

Sushumna, one of the three most important nadis, is the central channel through which life force flows (*nadi* means "stream"). A feeling is experienced as pranic energy passes upward, similar to that felt when engaging the bandhas. The other two important nadis are *ida* and *pingala*, the left and right channels along the spine.

Chakras

The Chakra System: The Cosmic Self

The *cakras* (Original spelling) come from an ancient tradition, the word appearing in India a few thousand years ago at the time of an invasion by Indo-European peoples (Aryans). This became known as the *Vedic* period, when a cultural mixing took place throughout India over the following centuries. The chakra was symbolically shown as a ring of light, with a historical meaning of "to bring in a new age." Chakras are mentioned in the *Vedas*, the ancient Hindu text of knowledge.

Though a mystery from the past, we know the Sanskrit word *chakra* itself means "wheel," as in the wheel of time, believed also to be a metaphor for the sun, therefore representing celestial balance. Yogic literature mentions the chakras as psychic centers of consciousness as early as 200 B.C. in Patanjali's *Yoga Sutras*. The chakras as energy centers became an integral part of yoga philosophy through the Tantric tradition in the seventh century A.D., where integration of the many forces of the universe was emphasized. Yoga began to incorporate the whole being.

There are seven basic chakras (other minor ones are in the extremities) that work together as a complete system, sometimes called the "inner organs of the esoteric (obscure) body," and which are found along the spine. They intersect with the nadis (spinal energy channels) as well as the endocrine system and nerve plexi. One could call the chakras "psychoenergetic"

centers. They link to the natural elements of earth, water, fire, air, and ether, and their qualities help define human purpose. They are believed to receive, digest, distribute, and transmit life energy and are hence known as the "seven roots of awakening."

The seven primary chakras are listed here, including the Sanskrit word for each. The sacred, ancient language of Sanskrit is revered as being designed for enlightenment, as are the chakras. The meaning and effects of the chakra system go way beyond what is indicated in this book—energy flow and auric fields are best described by other experts such as Barbara Brennan and Cyndi Dale. The text *Yoga and Psychotherapy* by Swami Rama is also useful and considered the authoritative work on Chakras.

1. Root Chakra—*Muladhara*
foundation; primal needs; grounding; connected; security
color: red; planet: Saturn; element: earth; sense: smell
location: above the anus, base of the spine, pelvic floor
governs feet, legs, large intestine, perineum
animal: elephant; root sound: *lam*
Kundalini Shakti coils here, power of the divine feminine

2. Sacral Chakra—*Svadhisthana*
womb; emotional/sex flow; sweetness; pleasure; creativity
color: orange; planet: Pluto/Moon; element: water; sense: taste
location: front face of lower spine, pelvis, sacrum
governs fertility, lower back and hips, bladder, kidneys, ovaries, testes
animal: crocodile; root sound: *vam*
expansion of one's own individuality

3. Solar Plexus Chakra—*Manipura*
gut feelings; breath; warrior (courage); brilliant jewel; personal power
color: yellow; planet: Sun/Mars; element: fire; sense: sight
location: solar plexus, union of diaphragm, psoas, organs, centered around the navel
governs digestion, metabolism, emotions, universality of life, pancreas, adrenal glands
animal: ram; root sound: *ram*
influences the immune, nervous, and muscular systems

4. Heart Chakra—*Anahata*
divine acceptance; love; relationships; passion;
joy of life
color: green/pink; planet: Venus; element: air;
sense: skin
location: upper chest, heart, lungs
governs upper back, psychic ability, some
emotions, openness to life, thymus gland
animal: antelope; root sound: *yam*
engulfs the rhythm of the universe

5. Throat Chakra—*Vishuddha*
communication; self-expression; harmony;
vibration; grace; dreams
color: sky blue; planet: Mercury/Jupiter; element:
space; sense: hearing
location: throat, neck, ears, mouth
governs sound, power of voice, assimilation,
thyroid and parathyroid glands
animal: white elephant; root sound: *ham*
*communicates inner truth to the world, ascends
physical to spiritual*

6. Brow Chakra—*Ajna*
third eye; intuition; concentration; conscience;
devotion; neutrality
color: indigo/purple; planet: Neptune; element:
light; sense: the mind
location: center of head between and above
eyebrows
governs creativity, imagination, understanding,
rational dreaming, pineal gland
animal: black antelope; root sound: *om*
provides opportunity to see everything as sacred

7. Crown Chakra—*Sahasrara*
pure consciousness; spirituality; true wisdom;
integration; bliss
color: white, also violet/gold; planet: Uranus/
Ketu; beyond elements
location: top of the head, cerebral cortex
governs all functions of the body and mind, other
chakras, pituitary gland
symbol: thousand-petaled lotus (void)
*Kundalini energy (Shakti) unites with male energy
(Shiva) to transcend into the essence of all*

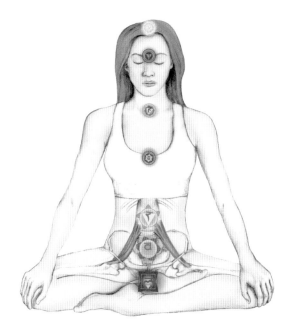

The Eight Limbs of Yoga

Throughout this text the limbs of yoga have been mentioned. They are listed here for reference, defined by Patanjali some 2500 years ago, as a guide for living the yogic way of life.

1. *Yamas* (restraints)
2. *Niyamas* (observances)
3. *Asanas* (postures)
4. *Pranayama* (mindful breathing)
5. *Pratyahara* (turning inward)
6. *Dharana* (concentration)
7. *Dhyana* (meditation)
8. *Samadhi* (bliss)

In this anatomical and movement text we are concerned mostly with the *asanas* (3) and *pranayama* (4), developing physical balance and breath through awareness.

Yoga is not a linear method. Practice is begun on the mat, learning techniques from different teachers. The complete teachings of yoga philosophy are discovered as one continues to delve into the essence of yoga as it is incorporated into daily life.

All things are connected.

79

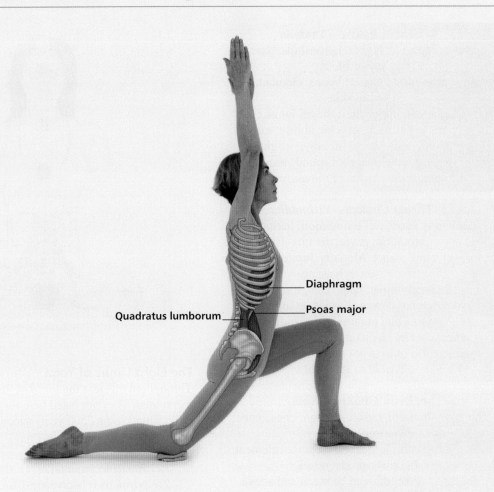

Diaphragm

Psoas major

Quadratus lumborum

Anjani = mother of Hanuma; (ahn-jan-ee-AHS-anna)

Awareness: Breath, stretch, strength, heart and hip opener, core work, balance, bandhas, *drishti*.

Action and Alignment: Spine extension, shoulder flexion, shoulder girdle upward rotation, hip flexion and extension, knee flexion, plantar flexion of back foot. Extend the back foot. Front knee is bent forward over the ankle, with the pelvis even.

Technique: From *Uttanasana*, hands on either side of the feet or on blocks, step back with one foot to a low lunge position. Bend the back knee to rest it on the floor; a blanket may be placed under the knee. Extend the back foot. Release the arms out and up, creating a crescent shape from the hips to the hands (slight backbend). Gaze is forward or up to the hands. This posture is included as a warm-up in Sun Salutation.

Helpful Hints: Lifting the pelvic floor and engaging the core will aid the balance in this posture. Drop the tailbone and press the shoulders and shoulder blades down. If possible, push the pelvis forward to create more stretch for the front of the back thigh. Place the hands on the front thigh, on the sacrum, or in Cactus if there is a shoulder problem.

Counter Pose: *Adho Mukha Svanasana* (see Chapter 6)

Muscles of the Shoulder and Upper Arm

This complex area is simplified by breaking it down into the following joint areas:

- The shoulder girdle—the sternoclavicular joint
- The shoulder joint—the glenohumeral joint
- The elbow joint—the humeroulnar joint

Each joint area has its own specific actions, and a few muscles share attachments across two or more different joints. These muscles are known as "multiarticulate" because they work more than one joint.

The structure of the shoulder permits a wide range of motion, allowing considerable freedom in the positioning of the arm and the hand. Movements of the shoulder region are determined by muscles located on the chest, back, and upper arms. The brachial plexus nerve center passes through here and down the arm, innervating many of the muscles of the entire arm.

Shoulder Girdle

Structure
This is a separate area that allows the shoulder joint to achieve an excellent range of motion of the arm. Three bones articulate in two different areas to form the shoulder girdle: the clavicle, scapula, and sternum. Movements of the shoulder girdle are activated mostly at the sternoclavicular joint, which in turn moves the scapula. This joint is the only point where the axial skeleton connects to the trunk. The lesser joints are the scapulothoracic, acromioclavicular, and coracoclavicular, where bones articulate but not much movement happens.

Actions
There are six to eight actions of the shoulder girdle joint, depending on which text is referred to. For the purposes of this book all movements are listed, as they are major actions associated with many yoga

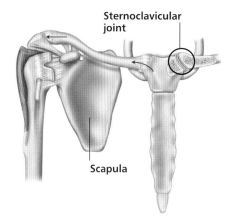

Sternoclavicular joint

Scapula

postures. They are elevation, depression, abduction (protraction) and adduction (retraction), upward and downward rotation, and forward and backward tilt. The actions are indicated by how the scapula moves in space: the scapula moving up is elevation, down is depression, away from the spine is abduction, and toward the spine adduction. Upward rotation is accomplished by the scapula's inferior angle moving out and up; downward rotation is the return from this position. Forward tilt is best seen when the arm is extended behind the body, and backward tilt can happen in a backbend, where the superior scapula tips posteriorly. Chapter 1 illustrates some of these actions.

Almost all yoga asanas incorporate shoulder girdle movement. Even in *Tadasana* (Mountain Pose) and sitting meditation, one is reminded to "slide the shoulder blades down the back." This is a subtle combination of the actions of adduction, downward rotation, and depression.

Muscles
The six muscles working the girdle are the pectoralis minor, serratus anterior, subclavius, levator scapula, rhomboids, and trapezius. All six are located on the chest (anterior) or upper back (posterior). Two of them, the levator scapula and the upper trapezius, are biarticulate with the cervical spine. Each muscle is very specific, especially the trapezius, as its different parts can do opposite actions, a rare occurrence in muscles.

LEVATOR SCAPULAE

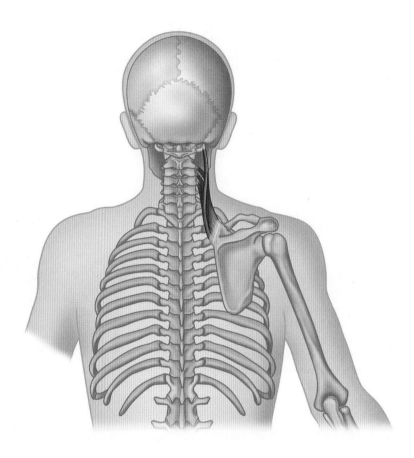

Latin, *levare*, to lift; *scapulae*, of the shoulder blade.

Levator scapulae is deep to sternocleidomastoideus and trapezius. It is named after its action of elevating the scapula.

Origin
Posterior tubercles of the transverse processes of the first three or four cervical vertebrae (C1–C4).

Insertion
Medial (vertebral) border of the scapula, between the superior angle and spine of the scapula.

Action
Elevates scapula. Helps retract scapula. Helps bend neck laterally.

Nerve
Dorsal scapular nerve, C4, C5, and cervical nerves, C3, C4.

Basic functional movement
Example: Carrying a heavy bag. Shoulder shrugs.

Movements that may injure this muscle
Sudden neck movement, such as whiplash. This muscle, along with the upper trapezius, is often tight because of stress; therefore, stretching is necessary.

Asanas that use this muscle[4]
Strengthening: *Makarasana*; Side Neck Bends. Shoulder Shrugs.
Stretching: Cervical Side Bends. Shoulder Rolls.

---

4   In any asana where the arm is raised, the shoulder girdle must also elevate to bring the arm past the horizontal to a vertical position. It is then its responsibility to do the reverse action, depression, to keep the shoulders down away from the ears.

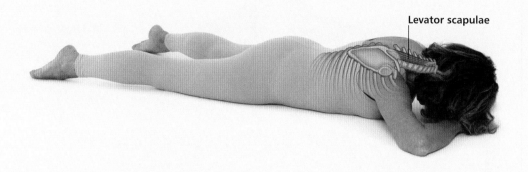

Levator scapulae

Makara = sea creature; (mak-ah-RAHS-ana)

Awareness: Breath, stretch, expansion, relaxation, release.

Actions and Alignment: Shoulder abduction, shoulder girdle elevation, elbow flexion, hip outward rotation, knee extension, ankle plantar flexion. Spine in neutral.

Technique: Lie on the belly (prone position), arms elevated with one hand on top of the other. Rest the forehead on the hands. Extend the body and position the feet mat-width apart, with the legs rotated out. Warm the body with the breath; engagement of the core, or even bandhas, can be done here.

Helpful Hints: This position is ideal at the beginning of class, or as a warm-up to Cobra and Locust. Awareness of breath and how the body responds on the inhale and exhale is deeply experienced through the support of the floor. The legs can rotate in if the feet are compromised. If lying on the belly is uncomfortable, one can turn over onto the back. A blanket can be rolled under the chest and shoulders for support; remember to keep the neck extended, not lifted.

Counter Pose: Table to *Balasana* (see Chapter 8).

TRAPEZIUS

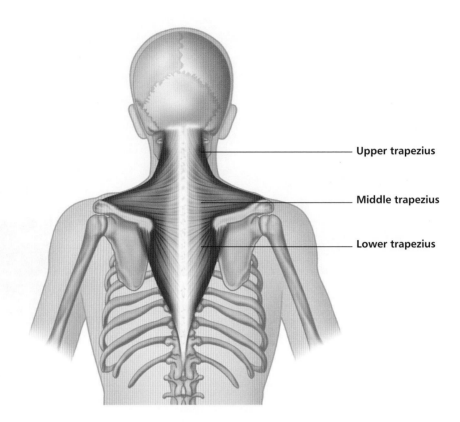

Upper trapezius

Middle trapezius

Lower trapezius

Greek, *trapezoeides*, table shaped.

The left and right trapezius viewed as a whole create a trapezium in shape, thus giving this muscle its name.

Origin
Medial third of superior nuchal line of occipital bone. External occipital protuberance. Ligamentum nuchae. Spinous processes and supraspinous ligaments of seventh cervical vertebra (C7) and all thoracic vertebrae (T1–T12).

Insertion
Posterior border of lateral third of clavicle. Medial border of acromion. Upper border of the crest of the spine of scapula and the tubercle on this crest.

Action
Upper fibers: Pull the shoulder girdle up (elevation). Help prevent depression of the shoulder girdle when a weight is carried on the shoulder or in the hand.
Middle fibers: Retract (adduct) the scapula.
Lower fibers: Depress the scapula, particularly against resistance, as when using the hands to get up from a chair.
Upper and lower fibers together: Rotate the scapula, as in elevating the arm above the head.

Nerve
Motor supply: Accessory XI nerve. Sensory supply (proprioception): Ventral ramus of cervical nerves, C2, C3, C4.

Basic functional movement
Retraction (adduction).
Example of upper and lower fibers working together: Painting a ceiling (upward rotation).

Movements that may injure this muscle
Falling (breaking a fall with the arms reaching out).

Asanas that heavily use this muscle
All asanas that incorporate the shoulder blades, whether in movement or stabilization.
Strengthening: *Salabhasana*, *Adho Mukha Svanasana*. *Urdhva Mukha Svanasana*. Plank. *Bhujangasana*. *Dhanurasana*. *Urdhva Dhanurasana* (Full Wheel).
Stretching: *Garudasana* (Eagle Arms). *Balasana* (Child's Pose, arms by sides). *Janu Sirsasana* (Head to Knee Forward Bend).

RHOMBOIDEUS MINOR

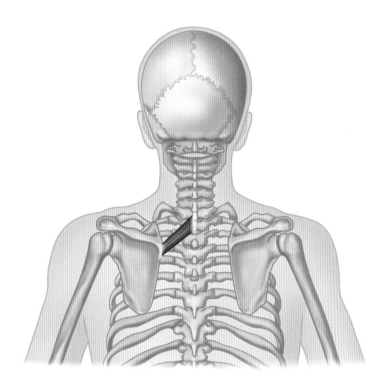

Greek, *rhomboeides*, parallelogram shaped, with opposite sides and angles equal. **Latin**, *minor*, smaller.

So named because of its shape.

Origin
Spinous processes and supraspinous ligaments of the seventh cervical and first thoracic vertebrae. Lower part of ligamentum nuchae.

Insertion
Medial (vertebral) border of scapula at the level of the spine of scapula.

Action
Retracts (adducts) and stabilizes scapula. Slightly elevates medial border of scapula, causing downward rotation (therefore depressing the lateral angle). Slightly assists in outer range adduction of arm (i.e., from arm overhead to arm at shoulder level).

Nerve
Dorsal scapular nerve, C4, C5.

Basic functional movement
Pulling something toward you, such as opening a drawer.

Asanas that heavily use this muscle
See list of asanas under "Rhomboideus Major."

RHOMBOIDEUS MAJOR

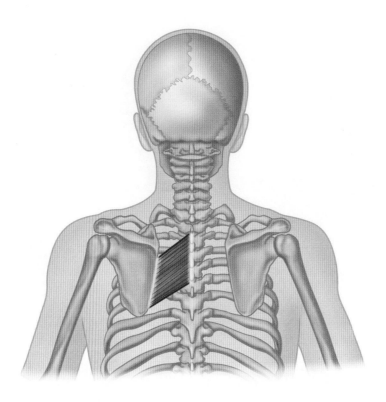

Greek, *rhomboeides*, parallelogram shaped, with opposite sides and angles equal. **Latin**, *major*, larger.

The rhomboideus major runs parallel to, and is often continuous with, the rhomboideus minor. It is so named because of its shape.

Origin
Spinous processes and supraspinous ligaments of second to fifth thoracic vertebrae (T2–T5).

Insertion
Medial border of the scapula, between the spine of the scapula and the inferior angle.

Action
Retracts (adducts) and stabilizes the scapula. Slightly elevates medial border of the scapula causing downward rotation. Slightly assists in outer range of adduction of arm (i.e., from arm overhead to arm at shoulder level).

Nerve
Dorsal scapular nerve, C4, C5.

Basic functional movement
Pulling something toward you, such as opening a drawer. Rhomboids are synergistic with each other, meaning the major and minor both do the same actions. They also work along with the trapezius in adduction.

Movements that may injure this muscle
Falling (breaking a fall with the arms reaching out).

Asanas that heavily use this muscle
All asanas that incorporate the shoulder blades, whether in movement or stabilization.
Strengthening: *Salabhasana. Urdhva Mukha Svanasana. Chaturanga Dandasana. Bhujangasana. Dhanurasana. Urdhva Dhanurasana. Virabhadrasana I, II, III.*
Stretching: *Utkatasana* (Chair, arms up). *Balasana* (Child's Pose). *Garudasana* (Eagle Arms).

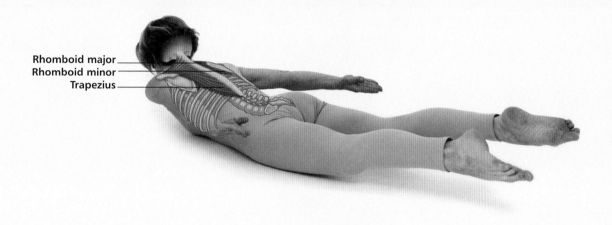

Rhomboid major
Rhomboid minor
Trapezius

salabha = grasshopper, locust;
(sha-lab-AHS-anna)

Awareness: Breath, lifting of heart, expansion of lungs, strength, stretch, stimulation of core, power.

Action and Alignment: Spine hyperextension, shoulder extension and inward rotation, shoulder girdle retraction, elbow and wrist extension, radioulnar supination, hip and knee extension, ankle plantar flexion. Core and leg engagement, head in line with the spine.

Technique: Lie on the belly, with the arms extended alongside the body, palms facing up, and forehead on the floor. Lift the torso, arms, and head up from the floor, with the hip bones grounded into the mat. The legs also extend and lift as the core is engaged to protect the lower back. The gaze is forward without crunching the cervical spine. The spinal extensors must contract to lift the upper body against gravity for full benefit, as the scapula retracts toward the spine. Deep breath work is needed as the posture is held.

Helpful Hints: Experience *Bhujangasana* as a warm-up, where the hands can be lifted off the floor to make sure the spinal extensors are doing the work. Once this is established, the full Locust can be done. This is a backbend and good warm-up for more advanced work. If the lumbar spine is compromised, separate the feet and engage the core more effectively. Some may wish to pad the hip bones with a blanket.

Counter Pose: *Balasana* (see Chapter 8).

SERRATUS ANTERIOR

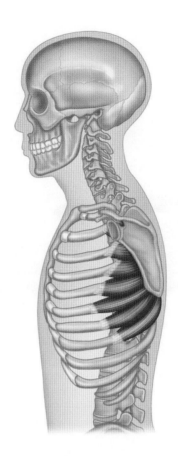

Latin, *serratus*, serrated; *anterior*, in front.

The serratus anterior forms the medial wall of the axilla, along with the upper five ribs. It is a large muscle composed of a series of finger-like slips. The lower slips interdigitate with the origin of the external oblique.

Origin
Outer surfaces and superior borders of upper eight or nine ribs and the fascia covering their intercostal spaces.

Insertion
Anterior (costal) surface of the medial border of scapula and inferior angle of scapula.

Action
Rotates scapula for abduction and flexion of arm. Protracts scapula (pulls it forward on the chest wall and holds it closely into the chest wall), facilitating pushing movements such as press-ups or punching.

Nerve
Long thoracic nerve, C5, C6, C7, C8.

Basic functional movement
Reaching forward for something barely within reach.

Movements that may injure this muscle
A lesion of the long thoracic nerve will result in the medial border of the scapula falling away from the posterior chest wall, causing a "winged scapula" (looking like an angel's wing). A weak muscle will also produce a winged scapula, especially when holding a weight in front of the body.

Asanas that heavily use this muscle
All asanas that incorporate the shoulder blades in stabilization.
Strengthening: *Adho Mukha Svanasana. Chaturanga Dandasana* (on way up). *Garudasana* (Eagle Arms). *Trikonasana*.
Stretching: Clasping hands behind the torso.

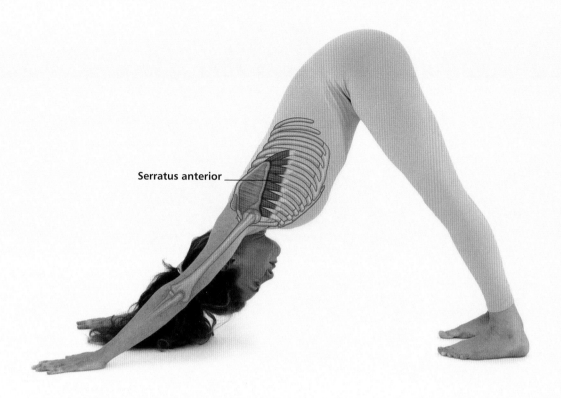

Serratus anterior

adho = downward; *mukha* = face; *svana* = dog; (ah-doh moo-kah svah-NAHS-anna)

Awareness: Breath, strength, stretch, calming, energizing, therapeutic for whole body.

Action and Alignment: Spine extension, shoulder flexion and outward rotation, shoulder girdle stabilization and upward rotation, elbow and wrist extension, hip and knee extension, ankle dorsiflexion. Body is in an inverted "V" position.

Technique: Begin in a Table position (on hands and knees), with the toes tucked under. Lift the knees and tailbone up as the core is engaged, and shift the weight of the body toward the legs. The arms are supportive, with the head in line with them. The heels move toward the floor, and the rib cage is relaxed.

Helpful Hints: This posture creates an intense stretch for the hamstrings in the back of the thighs. Relaxing the knees will ease the strain of tight hamstrings (Chapter 8). Moving the shoulders outward and down away from the ears will create more support and ease the effort of the arms. Hold the asana for at least three full breaths, and relax. The concept of "spiraling" can be discovered here—from the thumbs to the outer elbows and shoulders, and from the big toes to the outer knees and hips. Down Dog is a great counter pose to many other asanas, and used as a rest during Sun Salutation series.

Counter Pose: *Balasana* (see Chapter 8).

PECTORALIS MINOR

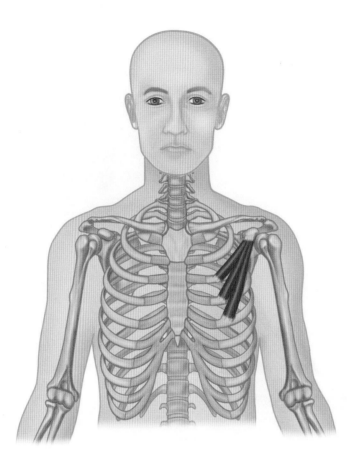

Latin, *pectoralis*, relating to the chest; *minor*, smaller.

Pectoralis minor is a flat triangular muscle lying posterior to, and concealed by, pectoralis major. Along with pectoralis major, it forms the anterior wall of the axilla.

Origin
Outer surfaces of third, fourth, and fifth ribs and fascia of the corresponding intercostal spaces.

Insertion
Coracoid process of scapula.

Action
Draws scapula forward and downward. Raises ribs during forced inspiration (it is an accessory muscle of inspiration when the scapula is stabilized by the rhomboids and trapezius).

Nerve
Medial pectoral nerve with fibers from a communicating branch of the lateral pectoral nerve, C6, C7, C8, T1.

Basic functional movement
Pushing on arms of chair to stand up. In yoga, reaching arms behind the back to clasp hands, then raising them. Also synergistic with serratus anterior in abduction.

Movements that may injure or compromise this muscle
Reaching far behind quickly. Often tight because of consistent frontal movements of the arms as in working at the computer. Because the pectoralis minor has the two different actions of forward tilt and abduction, it is confusing as to when it is strengthening vs. stretching. Most importantly it needs to stretch.

Asanas that heavily use this muscle
Strengthening: Reverse Table. High *Chaturanga* (Plank). *Chaturanga Dandasana*. *Purvottanasana* (Reverse Plank). *Gomukasana*, bottom arm (all asanas where the arms reach behind the body in shoulder joint extension, causing forward tilt of scapula).
Stretching: Clasping hands behind the torso. *Gomukasana* (Cow Face).

SUBCLAVIUS

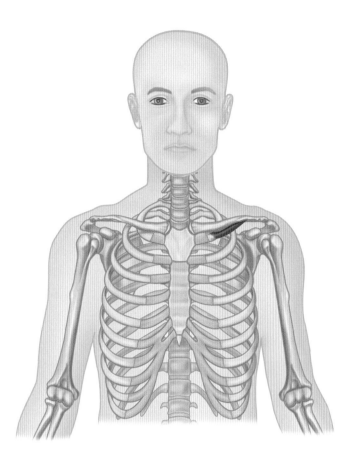

Latin, *sub*, under; *clavis*, key.

This muscle is posterior to, and concealed by, the clavicle and pectoralis major. Paralysis of this muscle produces no apparent effect.

Origin
Junction of the first rib and first costal cartilage.

Insertion
Floor of a groove on the lower (inferior) surface of the clavicle.

Action
Depresses clavicle and draws it toward the sternum, thereby steadying the clavicle in movements of the shoulder girdle.

Nerve
Nerve to subclavius, C5, C6.

Movements that may injure this muscle
Sudden impact to collar bone area. Unstable shoulder joint.

Asanas that heavily use this muscle
All asanas that require stabilization of the clavicle, especially arm supported postures.

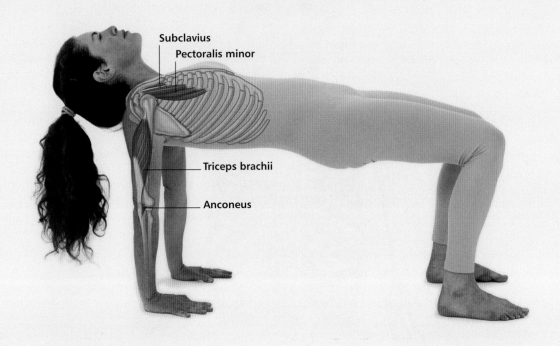

Subclavius

Pectoralis minor

Triceps brachii

Anconeus

ardha = half; *purva* = front, east; *ut* = intense; *tan* = extend; (ARD-hah PUR-voh-tan-AHS-anna)

Awareness: Breath, strength, stretch, shoulder and hip opener, pelvic stability, support.

Action and Alignment: Shoulder extension and inward rotation, shoulder girdle retraction, elbow and wrist/hand extension, core stabilization, hip extension, knee flexion. Spine neutral, wrists under shoulders, feet under knees.

Technique: From a sitting position with the legs in front and the knees bent, place the arms behind on the floor, fingers facing forward, and press the pelvis up in line with the shoulders and hips. The gaze is up toward the sky—do not drop the head back. This posture can be done at any time the front of the hips needs to open.

Helpful Hints: This is an intense stretch for the front of the shoulder and hips. Place the hips on a block for more support and less strain. If carpal tunnel syndrome is an issue, make a fist with the hands for stability.

Counter Pose: *Sukhasana, Dandasana.*

Shoulder Joint

Structure

The main shoulder joint is the glenohumeral joint, specifically the articulation between the scapula and the humerus. A multiaxial ball-and-socket joint, the structure comprises the glenoid cavity (socket) of the scapula, in which the head of the humerus (ball) sits. This cavity, or fossa, is shallow compared with other ball-and-socket joints, thus allowing greater range of motion, but less stability. The shoulder joint is complicated and multifaceted.

Connective Tissue

The head of the humerus is large in relation to the cavity it fits into. To achieve a tighter fit there is a fibro-cartilaginous ring called the "glenoid labrum" that helps seal the humerus in place more snugly. The shoulder joint capsule is also strengthened by means of the ligamentum semicirculare humeri, a ligamentous tissue that lies in close relationship with the tendons of the rotator cuff to bring integrity to the area.

Because the shoulder joint articulation is not deep and gravity acts as a force on the humerus, the ligaments of the joint must be very strong and intact to help hold the joint together. Three glenohumeral ligaments in the front of the joint and an inferior and superior coracohumeral ligament (running from the coracoid to the humerus) are the main reinforcing structures.

Actions

The upper arm (humerus) is the visual indicator when deciphering what action is happening (e.g., the upper arm in front of the body indicates flexion of the shoulder joint). The main actions are the true ball-and-socket joint actions of flexion, extension, abduction, adduction, and internal (medial) and external (lateral) rotation. Because the joint is so mobile (thanks to the aid of the shoulder girdle joint area), the joint can also hyperflex, hyperextend, hyperabduct, and hyperadduct. Add another true joint action of moving the humerus from the frontal to the sagittal plane and back again, and horizontal adduction/abduction is included. Diagonal movements are the combination of some of these actions. (Note: the action of horizontal adduction is sometimes called "horizontal flexion"; the action of horizontal abduction is also referred to as "horizontal extension"—see Chapter 1 for illustrations.)

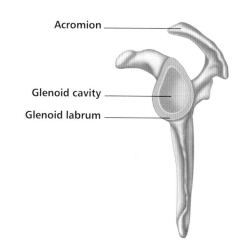

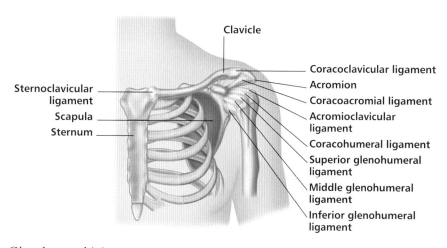

Glenohumeral joint.

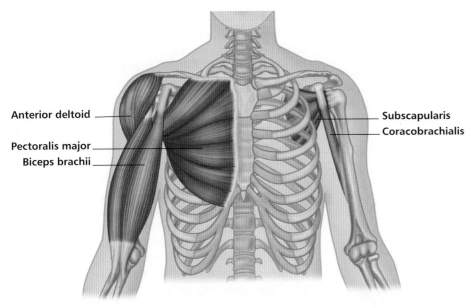

Anterior deltoid

Pectoralis major

Biceps brachii

Subscapularis

Coracobrachialis

Muscles that cross the shoulder joint (anterior view).

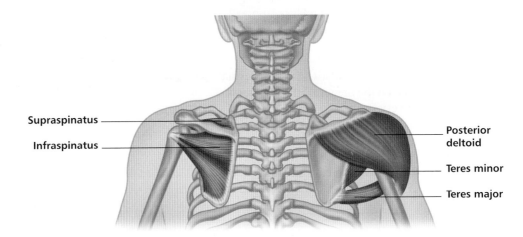

Supraspinatus

Infraspinatus

Posterior deltoid

Teres minor

Teres major

Muscles that cross the shoulder joint (posterior view).

Muscles

Muscles that move the upper arm have to cross the glenohumeral joint in order to work it. This is a major principle of kinesiology: if a muscle does not attach and then cross from one of the articulated bones to the other in some way, how can the bones be moved when the muscle is contracted?

Example: The infraspinatus muscle (see page 103) crosses the shoulder joint from the scapula to the humerus to work it. As it contracts concentrically (shortens), the arm is pulled backward and can rotate externally.

Viewed anteriorly, the muscles that cross the shoulder joint are the pectoralis major, anterior deltoid, coracobrachialis, and biceps brachii. The posterior muscles are the supraspinatus, infraspinatus, teres

major and minor, latissimus dorsi, posterior deltoid, and triceps brachii. The subscapularis rounds out the shoulder joint's 11 muscles (counting all deltoids as one muscle). Hidden behind the rib cage and on the anterior side of the scapula, the subscapularis is one of the four rotator cuff muscles of the shoulder joint (the "SITS muscles": supraspinatus, infraspinatus, teres minor, subscapularis).

To make things simpler, most of the time the anterior muscles do all forward movement, such as flexion, internal rotation, and horizontal adduction. Posterior-located muscles do the opposite actions of extension, external rotation, and horizontal abduction.

PECTORALIS MAJOR

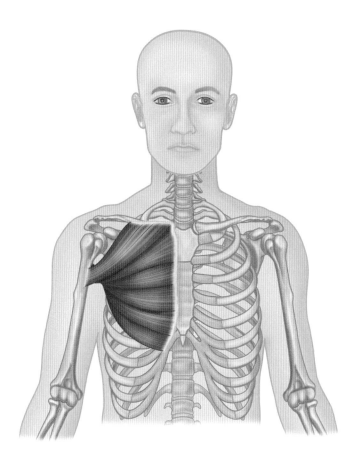

Latin, *pectoralis*, relating to the chest; *major*, larger.

Along with pectoralis minor, pectoralis major forms the anterior wall of the axilla.

Origin
Clavicular head: Medial half or two-thirds of front of clavicle. Sternocostal portion: Front of manubrium and body of sternum. Upper six costal cartilages. Rectus sheath.

Insertion
Crest below greater tubercle of humerus. Lateral lip of intertubercular sulcus (bicipital groove) of humerus.

Action
Adducts and medially rotates the humerus.
Clavicular portion: Flexes and medially rotates the shoulder joint and horizontally adducts the humerus toward the opposite shoulder.

Sternocostal portion: Obliquely adducts the humerus toward the opposite hip.
The pectoralis major is one of the main climbing muscles, pulling the body up to the fixed arm.

Nerve
Nerve to upper fibers: Lateral pectoral nerve, C5, C6, C7.
Nerve to lower fibers: Lateral and medial pectoral nerves, C6, C7, C8, T1.

Basic functional movement
Clavicular portion: Brings arm forward and across the body, such as in applying deodorant to opposite armpit.
Sternocostal portion: Pulling something down from above, such as a rope in bell ringing.
In yoga, supporting any arm balance.

Movements that may injure this muscle
Overuse. Lifting heavy weights.

Asanas that heavily use this muscle
Strengthening: High *Chaturanga* (Plank). *Chaturanga Dandasana*. *Garudasana* (Eagle Arms). *Bakasana* (Crow Pose). *Mayurasana* (Peacock).
Stretching: Reaching arms behind horizontally. *Gomukasana* (Cow Face).

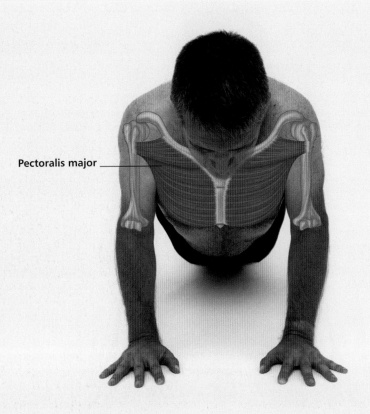

Pectoralis major

chatur = four; *anga* = limb; *danda* = staff; (chah-tur-angh-uh dahn-DAHS-ana)

Awareness: Breath, strength, stabilization, endurance, core, power.

Action and Alignment: Spine extension, shoulder flexion, shoulder girdle stabilization, elbow and wrist extension, core and pelvic stabilization, knee extension, ankle dorsiflexion. Body is in a straight horizontal line from head to feet.

Technique: From *Uttanasana*, step back with both feet to a push-up position. Hold for a few powerful breaths, engaging the core deeply. Keep the hands under the shoulders and lower down to the mat slowly while bending the elbows in toward the ribs. This movement is popular in *vinyasas* (flow of breath-synchronized postures) and Sun Salutation. High Plank variations include lifting one leg off the ground, or bringing one knee to the chest for more of a challenge.

Helpful Hints: This is a challenging pose for the entire body, and specifically targets the core. While in High Plank, lower the knees to the ground for more support. One can also bring the forearms to the ground, especially if there is a shoulder or wrist problem. The pectoralis major contracts in all phases: isometrically in High Plank and eccentrically on the way down (*Chaturanga*). If one attempts the most challenging movement, it contracts concentrically on the way back up from the floor. Gravity and body weight are the strong resisters.

Counter Pose: *Adho Mukha Svanasana.*

LATISSIMUS DORSI

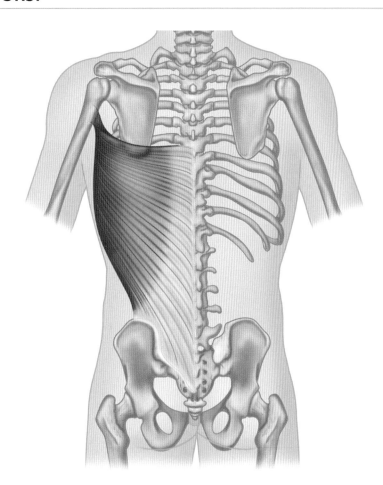

Latin, *latissimus*, widest; *dorsi*, of the back.

Along with subscapularis and teres major, the latissimus dorsi forms the posterior wall of the axilla.

Origin
Thoracolumbar fascia, which is attached to the spinous processes of the lower six thoracic vertebrae and all the lumbar and sacral vertebrae (T7–S5) and to the intervening supraspinous ligaments. Posterior part of iliac crest. Lower three or four ribs. Inferior angle of the scapula.

Insertion
Floor of the intertubercular sulcus (bicipital groove) of humerus.

Action
Extends the flexed arm. Adducts and medially rotates the humerus. It is one of the chief climbing muscles, since it pulls the shoulders downward and backward and pulls the trunk up to the fixed arms (thus also active in crawl swimming stroke). Assists in forced inspiration, by raising the lower ribs.

Nerve
Thoracodorsal nerve, C6, C7, C8, from the posterior cord of the brachial plexus.

Basic functional movement
Pushing on the arms of a chair to stand up. In yoga, supporting any arm balance.

Movements that may injure this muscle
Pulling a heavy weight down, or holding too heavy a weight out to the side.

Asanas that heavily use this muscle
Strengthening: *Urdhva Mukha Svanasana* (Up Dog). *Vasisthasana* (Side Plank). Stabilizing: High *Chaturanga* (Plank). *Chaturanga Dandasana*.
Stretching: *Adho Mukha Svanasana* (Down Dog). *Balasana* (Child's Pose). *Utkatasana* (Chair, with arms up).

TERES MAJOR

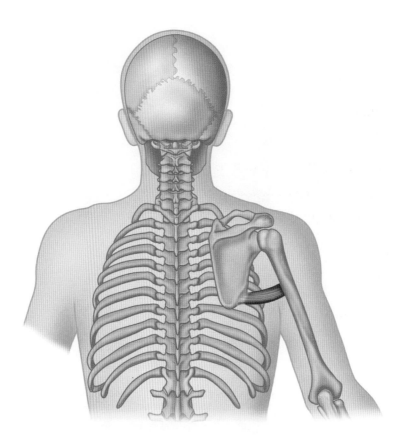

Latin, *teres*, rounded, finely shaped; *major*, larger.

The teres major together with the tendon of latissimus dorsi (which passes around it) and the subscapularis form the posterior fold of the axilla.

Origin
Oval area on the lower third of the posterior surface of the lateral border of the scapula.

Insertion
Medial lip of the intertubercular sulcus (bicipital groove) of humerus.

Action
Adducts humerus. Medially rotates humerus. Extends humerus from the flexed position.

Nerve
Lower subscapular nerve, C5, C6, C7, from the posterior cord of the brachial plexus.

Basic functional movement
Reaching into your back pocket.

Movements that may injure this muscle
See latissimus dorsi (page 97).

Asanas that heavily use this muscle
Synergistic with latissimus dorsi, so the same asanas apply.

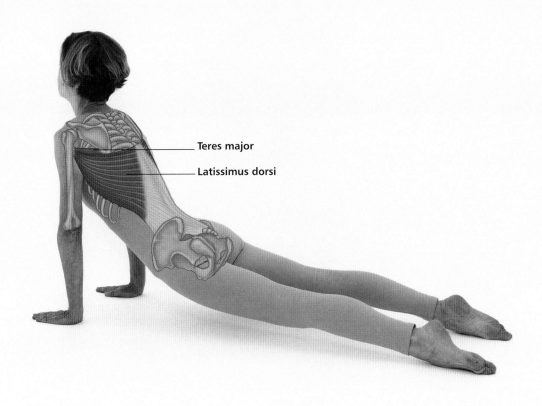

Teres major

Latissimus dorsi

urdhva = upward; *mukha* = face; *svana* = dog; (urd-vah moo-kah svan-AHS-anna)

Awareness: Breath, strength, stretch, support, core and pelvic stability, stimulation, openness.

Action and Alignment: Spine hyperextension, shoulder extension, shoulder girdle downward rotation, elbow and wrist extension, hip and knee extension, ankle plantar flexion. Hands are under the shoulders, and the legs are together.

Technique: From *Chaturanga Dandasana*, lift the torso forward and up into a backbend position. This is a strong movement for the arms and shoulders. The gaze is straight ahead, and the shoulders press down away from the ears. The legs and feet extend from the pelvis; a strong lift of the pelvic floor will help to engage the lower abdominals as well. This posture is added to Sun Salutation as a more challenging movement.

Helpful Hints: The lift of the sternum (breastbone) becomes what is generally termed a "heart-opener," as the front of the chest expands. Using a blanket under the thighs, or resting the knees on the floor, will aid the lower back as the core engages. Press the tops of the feet into the floor to energize the legs.

Counter Pose: *Adho Mukha Svanasana*.

DELTOIDEUS

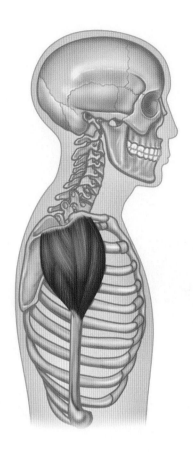

Greek, *deltoeides*, shaped like the Greek letter delta (resembling a triangle).

The deltoid muscle is composed of three parts: anterior, middle, and posterior. Only the middle part is multipennate, probably because its mechanical disadvantage of abduction of the shoulder joint requires extra strength.

Origin
Anterior fibers: Anterior border and superior surface of the lateral third of the clavicle.
Middle fibers: Lateral border of the acromion process.
Posterior fibers: Lower lip of the crest of the spine of the scapula.

Insertion
Deltoid tuberosity, situated halfway down the lateral surface of the shaft of the humerus.

Action
Anterior fibers: Flex and medially rotate the humerus.
Middle fibers: Abduct the humerus at the shoulder joint (only after the movement has been initiated by supraspinatus).
Posterior fibers: Extend and laterally rotate the humerus.

Nerve
Axillary nerve, C5, C6, from the posterior cord of the brachial plexus.

Basic functional movement
Reaching for something out to the side. Raising the arm to wave. Deltoids are also strong stabilizers in arm balances.

Movements that may injure this muscle
Holding too heavy a weight out to the side. Overdoing swimming strokes or throwing movements.

Asanas that heavily use this muscle
Strengthening: *Vasisthasana* (Side Plank). Reverse Swan Dive from *Surya Namaskara*. *Virabhadrasana II* (Warrior II). *Trikonasana* (Triangle Pose). *Adho Mukha Svanasana* (posterior deltoid). Cactus Arms. Arm Balances.
Stretching: Arm Circles. Clasping hands in front and behind the back. Swan Dive in Sun Salutation.

Although most would not consider *Uttanasana* (see opposite) a deltoid-working pose, it does strengthen the anterior deltoid and stretch the posterior deltoid when the hands reach and press into the floor or a block. This asana is better known for its hip flexion movement as one hinges forward from the hip joint, as well as for using the hip and spinal extensor muscles, which contract to lift the torso back up. This is also discussed in Chapter 8.

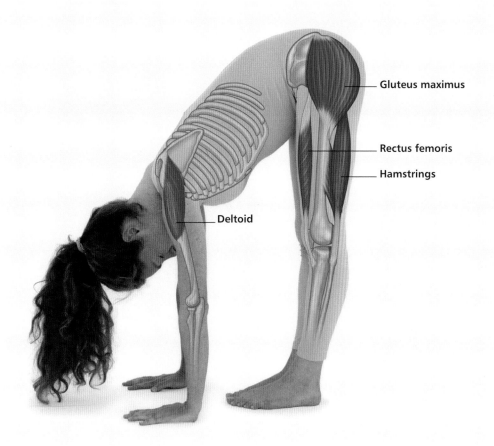

Gluteus maximus

Rectus femoris

Hamstrings

Deltoid

ut = intense; *tan* = stretch, extend; (oo-tan-AHS-anna)

Awareness: Breath, stretch, strength, length, calming, therapeutic, improves digestion, stimulation.

Action and Alignment:
Spinal extension, shoulder girdle stabilization, shoulder joint flexion, hip flexion, knee extension. Hips, knees, and ankle are in line with each other, with the weight of the torso felt directly over the center of the feet.

Technique: From *Tadasana*, prepare by lifting the arms high, then folding forward (Swan Dive) from the hips toward the ground. Think of the pelvis moving forward out over the legs. Place your hands on a block or the floor in front of the body and allow the spine to extend, head in line with the spine. Soften or even bend the knees so they do not lock back through the entire posture. Once this position is accomplished, one can begin to fold toward the legs into slight spine flexion (see advanced insert on the image).

Helpful Hints: This posture is ideal for warming up and transitions, as well as for incorporation into Sun Salutation. It is a great stretch for the hamstrings, gluteal muscles, and spinal extensors, but also a strength move for each of these muscle groups as the body is raised back up against gravity.

Counter Pose: *Tadasana*.

Rotator Cuff

The rotator cuff is composed of the supraspinatus, infraspinatus, teres minor, and subscapularis, commonly known as the "SITS muscles." The tendons of the "cuff" help hold the head of the humerus in contact with the glenoid cavity (fossa, socket) of the scapula during movements of the shoulder, thus helping to prevent dislocation of the joint. If dislocation occurs, the cuff is extremely compromised, overstretched, or possibly torn. Because the socket of the joint is shallow, the ligaments and tendons of the rotator cuff need to be strong enough to hold the humerus in place.

The following muscles will be demonstrated in one asana, *Gomukasana*, at the end of the section.

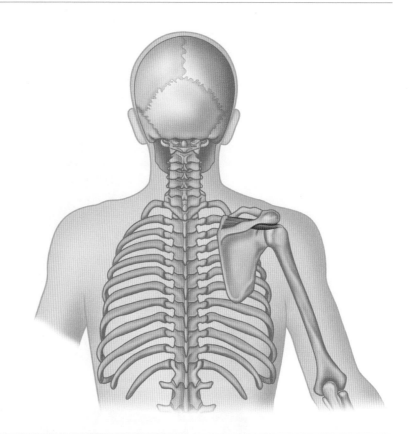

Latin, *supra*, above; *spina*, spine.

Origin
Supraspinous fossa of scapula.

Insertion
Upper aspect of the greater tubercle of the humerus. Capsule of shoulder joint.

Action
Initiates the process of abduction at the shoulder joint, so that the deltoid can take over in the later stages of abduction.

Nerve
Suprascapular nerve, C4, C5, C6, from the upper trunk of the brachial plexus.

Basic functional movement
Holding a shopping bag away from the side of the body. (Synergistic with the middle deltoid.)

Movements that may injure this muscle
Overuse. This is the most common muscle injured in the rotator cuff, because of its location and path.

Asanas that heavily use this muscle
Strengthening: *Gomukhasana* (Cow Face, both strengthening and stretching). *Vasisthasana* (Side Plank). Reverse Swan Dive from *Surya Namaskara*. *Virabhadrasana II* (Warrior II).
Stretching: Arm Circles. Swan Dive in Sun Salutation. Shoulder horizontal adduction.

INFRASPINATUS

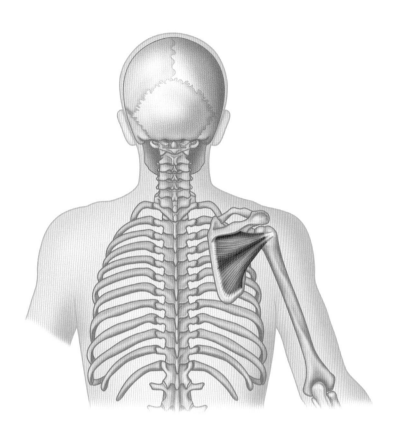

Latin, *infra*, below; *spina*, spine.

Origin
Infraspinous fossa of the scapula.

Insertion
Middle facet on the greater tubercle of humerus. Capsule of shoulder joint.

Action
As a rotator cuff, helps prevent posterior dislocation of the shoulder joint. Laterally rotates humerus.

Nerve
Suprascapular nerve, C4, C5, C6, from the upper trunk of the brachial plexus.

Basic functional movement
Brushing back of hair.

Movements that may injure this muscle
Excessive outward rotation of shoulder joint, as in swimming backstroke.

Asanas that heavily use this muscle
Gomukhasana. Adho Mukha Svanasana. Reverse Plank.
Stretching: Arm Circles. Rotating shoulders inward, such as Reverse Cactus.

TERES MINOR

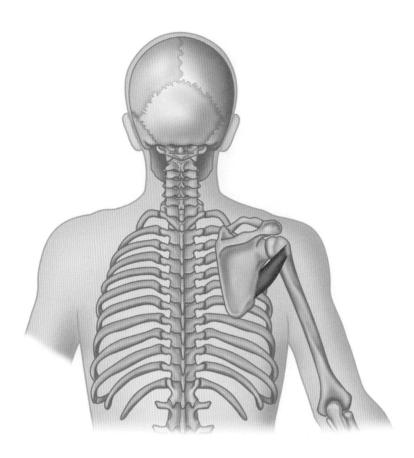

Latin, *teres*, rounded, finely shaped; *minor*, smaller.

Origin
Upper two-thirds of the lateral border of the dorsal surface of scapula.

Insertion
Lower facet on the greater tubercle of humerus. Capsule of shoulder joint.

Action
As a rotator cuff muscle, teres minor helps prevent upward dislocation of the shoulder joint. Laterally rotates humerus. Weakly adducts humerus. Synergistic with teres minor, so same actions apply.

Nerve
Axillary nerve, C5, C6, from the posterior cord of the brachial plexus.

Basic functional movement
Brushing back of hair.

Movements that may injure this muscle
Excessive outward rotation of shoulder joint.

Asanas that heavily use this muscle
See infraspinatus (page 103).

SUBSCAPULARIS

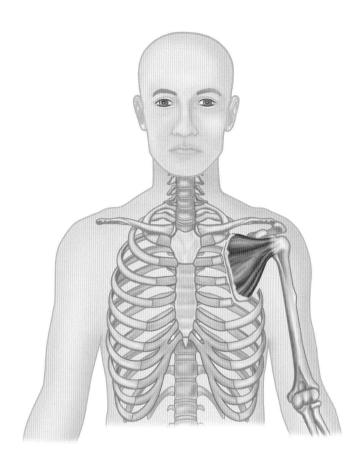

Latin, *sub*, under; *scapula*, shoulder blade.

The subscapularis constitutes the greater part of the posterior wall of the axilla.

Origin
Subscapular fossa and the groove along the lateral border of the anterior surface of scapula.

Insertion
Lesser tubercle of humerus. Capsule of shoulder joint.

Action
As a rotator cuff muscle, subscapularis stabilizes the glenohumeral joint, mainly preventing the head of the humerus from being pulled upward by the deltoid, biceps brachii, and long head of triceps brachii. Medially rotates humerus.

Nerve
Upper and lower subscapular nerves, C5, C6, C7, from the posterior cord of the brachial plexus.

Basic functional movement
Reaching into your back pocket.

Movements that may injure this muscle
Excessive inward rotation of the shoulder.

Asanas that heavily use this muscle
Gomukasana (Cow Face). Any asana that is supported by the arms, as the rotator cuff stabilizes. *Bakasana* (Crow/Crane Pose). Cactus Arms. Plank.
Stretching: Arms out and behind with palms facing up.

CORACOBRACHIALIS

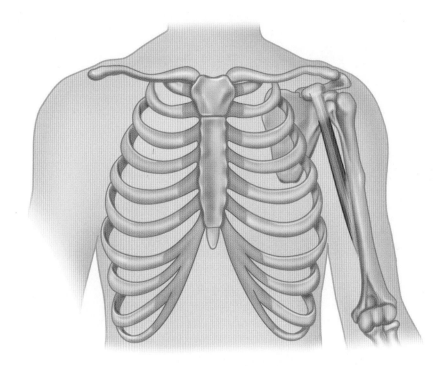

Greek, *korakoeides*, raven-like.
Latin, *brachialis*, relating to the arm.

The coracobrachialis is so named because it resembles a raven's beak. Along with the short head of biceps brachii and the humerus, it forms the lateral wall of the axilla. This is not considered a rotator cuff muscle; its actions are more synergistic with the short head of the biceps, but similar to those of the rotator cuff because of its stabilizing role.

Origin
Tip of the coracoid process of scapula.

Insertion
Medial aspect of humerus at mid-shaft.

Action
Weakly adducts shoulder joint. Possibly assists in flexion of shoulder joint. Helps stabilize humerus.

Nerve
Musculocutaneous nerve, C6, C7.

Basic functional movement
Mopping the floor. Mainly a stabilizer more than a "mover," aiding the rotator cuff.

Asanas that heavily use this muscle
Stabilizing asanas for rotator cuff will apply here.

Note: The biceps brachii and triceps brachii are also shoulder joint muscles, but associated more with the elbow joint. They are discussed in depth in the next section.

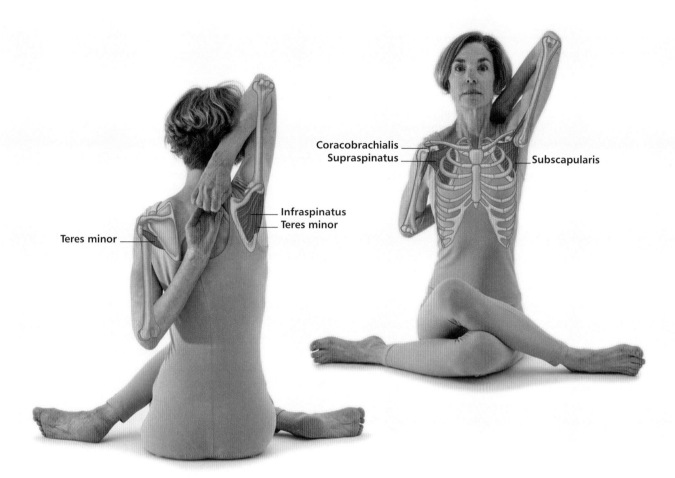

Teres minor

Coracobrachialis
Supraspinatus

Subscapularis

Infraspinatus
Teres minor

go = cow; *mukha* = face; (go-moo-KAHS-anna)

Awareness: Breath, stretch, chest expansion, core engagement, flexibility, *drishti*, concentration.

Action and Alignment: Spine extension, shoulder adduction, inward (bottom arm) and outward (top arm) rotation, shoulder girdle upward-and-downward rotation, elbow flexion, hip flexion/ adduction/outward rotation, knee flexion, ankle supination. Forearms are ideally in line with the spine, and the top knee is directly above the bottom knee.

Technique: From a sitting position, bend one leg under the other, actively aligning the knees one on top of the other, with the feet out to the sides. Keep the torso weight directly above the sit bones, engaging the pelvic floor and core. Reach one arm out and up, then bend at the elbow and place the palm of the hand on the upper spine. The other arm reaches behind the back, as the elbow bends and the hand extends up toward the top fingers. Whichever leg is on top, the opposite arm is the upward one.

Helpful Hints: This posture is difficult for both the arms and the hips, so it is best to do it after some good stretching and opening poses. Practice the asana diligently to improve flexibility without forcing. Holding a strap between the hands is beneficial for the arms. The legs can be positioned in *Sukhasana*, or one can even sit in a chair if the hips are tight. This pose is contraindicated if there are shoulder, hip, or knee problems.

Counter Pose: Repeat on the other side, then do a gentle twist in *Baddha Konasana* (see Chapter 8).

Elbow Joint

Structure
Technically called the "humeroulnar joint," the elbow joint is composed of the humerus (upper arm bone), radius, and ulna. The last two are the forearm bones, with the ulna being the most medial (pinky side). At the distal end of the humerus are the trochlea and the capitulum, which together form part of the elbow joint with the radius and ulna.

Actions
The elbow joint is a classic hinge (ginglymus) joint, where only two actions are performed: flexion (bending) and extension (straightening). These actions can only happen in the sagittal plane (anatomical position). Some people are able to hyperextend, or go beyond extension; this is contraindicated in yoga postures of arm support and balance and should be monitored.

Ligaments
Ligaments and muscles work together to provide stability and mobility to the joint. The importance of this fact cannot be overestimated in yoga asanas, as all joints need to be strong, yet flexible: "ease in balance with effort."

In the elbow, the ulnar (medial) collateral ligament consists of three strong bands (the anterior oblique, posterior oblique, and transverse oblique) that reinforce the medial side of the articular capsule. The radial (lateral) collateral ligament is a strong triangular ligament that reinforces the lateral side of the articular capsule. These ligaments connect the humerus to the ulna and act together to stabilize the elbow.

Muscles
Located on the upper and lower arm, with the proximal attachment above the joint, the main anterior muscles of the elbow are the biceps brachii, brachialis, and brachioradialis. The posterior muscles are the triceps brachii and the anconeus. The tendons of these muscles also act as stabilizers, crossing the elbow joint, and therefore provide extra security. It is easy to determine the action of the muscles: the flexors are anterior (anatomical position), and the extensors are posterior. Some of the extrinsic muscles in the forearm can also aid flexion, but since the contraction is weak, they will not be listed here.

The terminology helps in deciphering the names and types of some of the muscles: "bi" = two; "tri" = three. The biceps brachii therefore translates as "two heads" and "of the arm"; the triceps brachii means "three heads" and "of the arm." As mentioned in the shoulder joint section, these two muscles cross both the elbow joint and the shoulder joint. The biceps brachii, however, is a triarticulate muscle, meaning that it acts across three joints—the proximal radioulnar joint (upper forearm), the elbow joint, and the shoulder joint.

On the following three pages you will find similarities between the main elbow flexors, and the asanas they are active in. The difference in the strength of their contraction appears when the forearm is either supinated or pronated in the movement (Chapter 7).

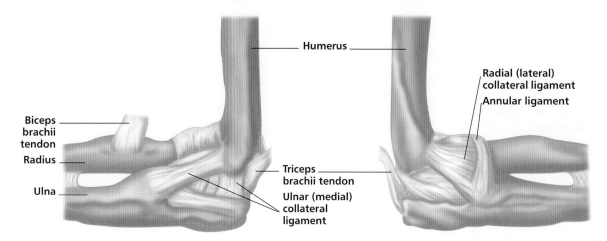

Humerus

Radial (lateral) collateral ligament

Annular ligament

Biceps brachii tendon

Radius

Ulna

Triceps brachii tendon

Ulnar (medial) collateral ligament

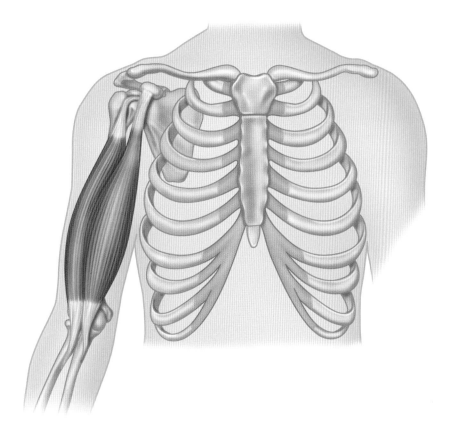

Latin, *biceps*, two-headed; *brachii*, of the arm.

Biceps brachii operates over three joints. It has two tendinous heads at its origin and two tendinous Insertions. Occasionally it has a third head, originating at the insertion of coracobrachialis. The short head forms part of the lateral wall of the axilla, along with the coracobrachialis and the humerus.

Origin
Short head: Tip of coracoid process of scapula.
Long head: Supraglenoid tubercle of scapula.

Insertion
Posterior part of radial tuberosity. Bicipital aponeurosis, which leads into the deep fascia on medial aspect of forearm.

Action
Flexes elbow joint. Supinates forearm. (It has been described as the muscle that puts in the corkscrew and pulls out the cork). Weakly flexes arm at the shoulder joint.

Nerve
Musculocutaneous nerve, C5, C6.

Basic functional movement
Example: Picking up an object. Bringing food to the mouth.

Movements that may injure this muscle
Lifting a heavy weight while bending the elbow. In yoga, lowering to the floor in *Chataranga Dandasana* incorrectly.

Asanas that heavily use this muscle
Strengthening: *Bakasana* (Crow Pose). Any forearm balance (Rabbit, Dolphin, *Sirsasana* [Headstand]).
Stretching: Clasping arms behind the body.

BRACHIALIS

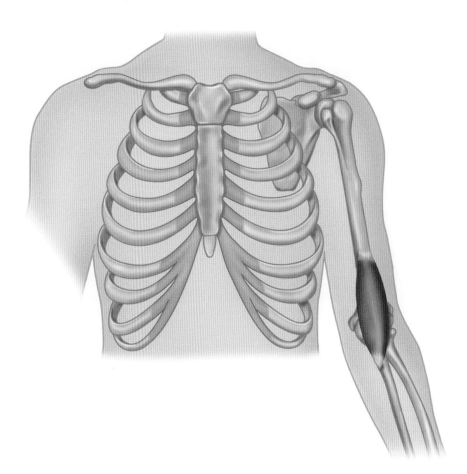

Latin, *brachialis*, relating to the arm.

Brachialis lies posterior to biceps brachii and is the main flexor of the elbow joint. Some fibers may be partly fused with the brachioradialis.

Origin
Lower (distal) two-thirds of anterior aspect of humerus.

Insertion
Coronoid process of ulna and tuberosity of ulna (i.e., area on front of upper part of shaft of ulna).

Action
Flexes elbow joint.

Nerve
Musculocutaneous nerve, C5, C6.

Basic functional movement
Example: Bringing food to the mouth.

Movements that may injure this muscle
Lifting a heavy weight while bending the elbow. In yoga, lowering to the floor in *Chataranga Dandasana* incorrectly.

Asanas that heavily use this muscle
Strengthening: *Bakasana* (Crow Pose). Any forearm balance (Rabbit, Dolphin, *Sirsasana* [Headstand]).
Stretching: Clasping arms behind the body.

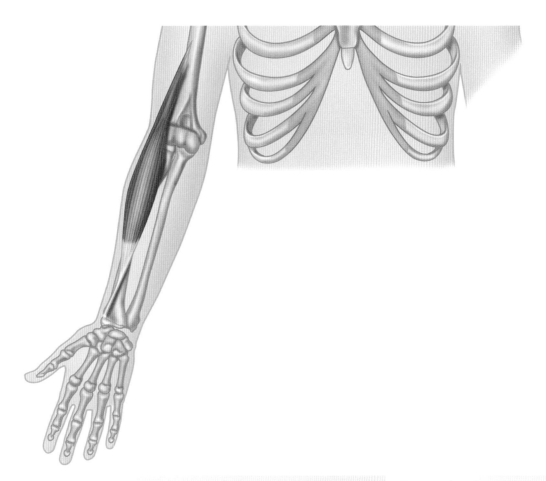

Latin, *brachium*, arm; *radius*, staff, spoke of wheel.

Part of the superficial group. The brachioradialis forms the lateral border of the cubital fossa. The muscle belly is prominent when working against resistance.

Origin
Upper two-thirds of the anterior aspect of lateral supracondylar ridge of humerus.

Insertion
Lower lateral end of radius, just above the styloid process.

Action
Flexes elbow joint. Assists in pronating and supinating forearm when these movements are resisted.

Nerve
Radial nerve, C5, C6.

Basic functional movement
Example: Turning a corkscrew.

Movements that may injure this muscle
Lifting a heavy weight while bending the elbow. In yoga, lowering to the floor in *Chataranga Dandasana* incorrectly.

Asanas that heavily use this muscle
Strengthening: *Bakasana* (Crow Pose). Any forearm balance (Rabbit, Dolphin, *Sirsasana* [Headstand]).
Stretching: Clasping arms behind the body.

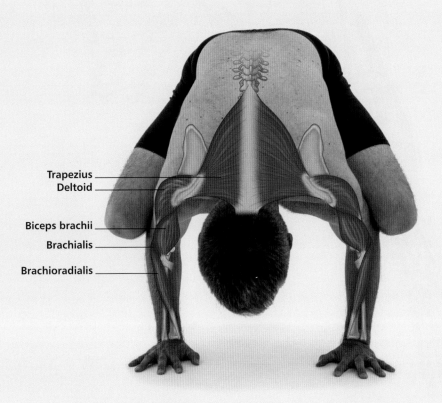

Trapezius

Deltoid

Biceps brachii

Brachialis

Brachioradialis

baka = crane; (bah-KAHS-anna)

Awareness: Breath, arm and core strength, balance.

Action and Alignment: Spine extension, shoulder and elbow flexion, wrist hyperextension, hip flexion and outward rotation, knee flexion, ankle plantar flexion. Spine is diagonal, with elbows above wrists.

Technique: From *Malasana* (squat), place the hands on the floor in front and under the shoulders, with the elbows bent and the knees on the triceps. Engaging the core, begin to lift the feet off the floor and toward each other as the arms support the body. The gaze is toward the front of the mat.

Helpful Hints: This posture is usually done toward the end of class after standing poses are completed. It would be wise to warm up the arms with *Chataranga Dandasana* first. The arms and wrists must be strong and the body balanced to hold *Bakasana*. A blanket placed in front on the mat is helpful if one tends to fall forward. Advanced variations are done with different leg positions.

Counter Pose: *Setu Bandhasana* (see Chapter 8).

TRICEPS BRACHII

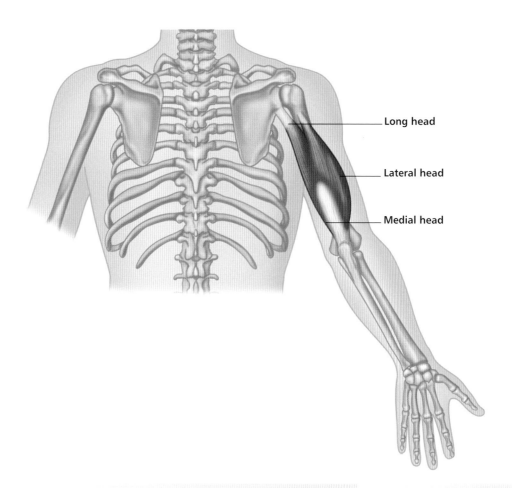

Long head
Lateral head
Medial head

Latin, *triceps*, three-headed; *brachii*, of the arm.

The triceps originates from three heads and is the only muscle on the back of the arm.

Origin
Long head: Infraglenoid tubercle of the scapula.
Lateral head: Upper half of posterior surface of shaft of humerus (above and lateral to the radial groove).
Medial head: Lower half of posterior surface of shaft of humerus (below and medial to the radial groove).

Insertion
Posterior part of the olecranon process of the ulna.

Action
Extends elbow joint. Long head can adduct the humerus and extend it from the flexed position. Stabilizes shoulder joint.

Nerve
Radial nerve, C6, C7, C8, T1.

Basic functional movement
Throwing objects. Pushing a door shut.

Movements that may injure this muscle
Pushing a heavy object away. Hyperextending the elbow. In yoga, Plank or *Purvottanasana* without support (see page 115).

Asanas that heavily use this muscle
All Plank positions (High, Side, Reverse). *Chaturanga Dandasana*. *Adho Mukha Vrksasana* (Handstand).
Stretching: *Garudasana* (Eagle Arms).

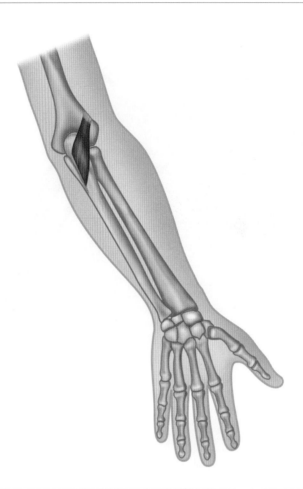

Latin, *anconeus*, of the elbow.

Origin
Posterior part of lateral epicondyle of humerus.

Insertion
Lateral surface of the olecranon process and upper portion of posterior surface of ulna.

Action
Assists triceps to extend forearm at elbow joint. May stabilize the ulna during pronation and supination.

Nerve
Radial nerve, C7, C8.

Basic functional movement
Pushing objects at arm's length.

Movements that may injure this muscle
Pushing a heavy object away. Hyperextending the elbow. In yoga, Plank or *Purvottanasana* without support.

Asanas that heavily use this muscle
All Plank positions (High, Side, Reverse). *Chaturanga Dandasana*. *Adho Mukha Vrksasana* (Handstand).
Stretching: *Garudasana* (Eagle Arms).

See *Ardha Purvottanasana* (Reverse Table) illustration under "Shoulder Girdle" section for triceps and anconeus. When the legs are straightened, the pose becomes *Purvottanasana*, explained on the following page.

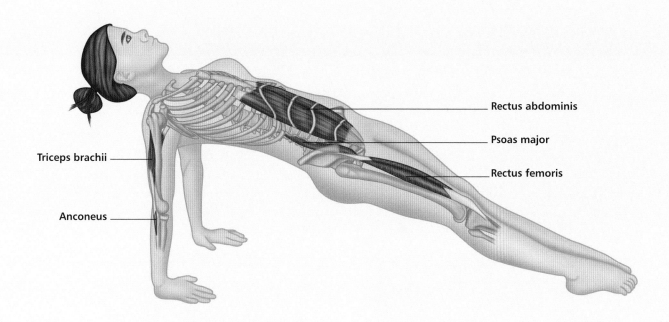

Rectus abdominis

Psoas major

Rectus femoris

Triceps brachii

Anconeus

purva = front; *ut* = intense; *tan* = stretch; (purr-vo-tah-NAHS-anna)

Awareness: Breath, strength, stretch, support, open shoulders and hips.

Action and Alignment:
Spine extension, shoulder hyperextension, shoulder girdle forward tilt, elbow and wrist extension, hip and knee extension, ankle plantar flexion. Body is in a horizontal line.

Technique: From *Dandasana*, place the hands behind the hips, with the fingers facing forward. Press the heels into the floor as the hips lift. The gaze is toward the sky.

Helpful Hints: If there is a shoulder problem, leave the hips on the floor and work more on gentle stretching of the front of the shoulder. This posture can be done at any time during class, especially after sitting for some time.

Counter Pose: *Dandasana* or any sitting forward bend.

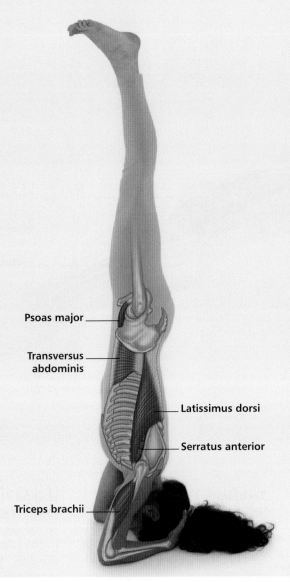

Psoas major

Transversus
abdominis

Latissimus dorsi

Serratus anterior

Triceps brachii

Summary for Upper Body Stabilization Muscles: The King of Asanas

sirsa = head; (shir-SHAHS-anna) Sometimes called *Salamba Sirsasana* (Supported Headstand).

Awareness: Breath, strength, balance, core, support, determination, calms the mind, stimulates glands, therapeutic.

Action and Alignment: Spine extension, shoulder flexion, shoulder girdle stabilization, elbow flexion, knee extension, ankle dorsiflexion or plantar flexion. Body is inverted vertically, with the pelvis/hips neutral.

Technique: From *Vajrasana* (see chapter 2), put the forearms on the floor, with the hands clasped and the elbows in. Place the back of the head into the palms and press firmly into the floor with the forearms so as not to put weight on the top of the head. Begin to lift the hips up and over the shoulders. Once balance is established with core engagement, straighten the legs to the sky.

Helpful Hints: *Note that care must be exercised in any inversion of the head if blood pressure has not been checked or if there are retinal eye conditions.* If a beginner, use the wall or another person for support. Go up and down slowly. A common correction is to soften the ribs and lengthen the lower back by pulling the core in. It is very difficult for some people to turn upside down. Once this is experienced, practice and determination will allow one to become more confident. Held for up to three minutes, this pose is best performed toward the end of class.

Counter Pose: *Setu Bandhasana* (see Chapter 8); Legs Up The Wall.

Muscles of the Forearm and Hand

The wrist and hand together comprise 27 bones, numerous ligaments, and many muscles and tendons. These components shape the forearm and are fundamental in developing the fine motor capabilities of the fingers. Remembering that the definition of a joint is the articulation between two bones, imagine how many joints are located in this area. The main joints associated with yoga will be discussed in this chapter.

Radioulnar Joint

Structure

The radioulnar joint is where the radius and ulna bones articulate with one another, both at the proximal end (near the elbow) and at the distal end (near the wrist). This is the rotary joint of the forearm, active in asanas such as Down Dog. Often confused with the elbow joint, the radioulnar joint is a separate joint, classified as a "pivot joint." It is uniaxial, working in the horizontal/transverse plane only.

Actions

Pronation and supination happen here. Supination is best described at this joint as the palm facing forward (anatomical position), also called "palm up." The radius externally rotates to a parallel position with the ulna. In pronation, the palm of the hand faces backward, or "palm down." The radius rotates internally so that it lies diagonally across the ulna.

Strengthening and stretching the muscles of this joint area is not as vital as making sure that the actions of pronation and supination are performed equally. For example, in *Virabhadrasana II*, the forearm position is pronation; adding the action of supination will allow the shoulder blades to settle and help access the entire shoulder area in a subtle yet positive way. The arms can then return to pronation as the practitioner experiences the difference.

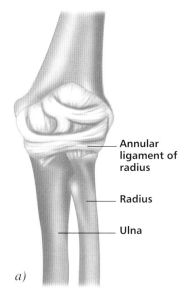

Annular ligament of radius

Radius

Ulna

a)

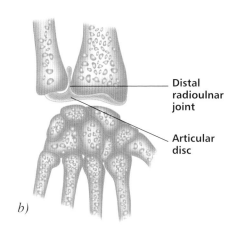

Distal radioulnar joint

Articular disc

b)

The radioulnar joint; a) proximal end, b) distal end.

PRONATOR TERES

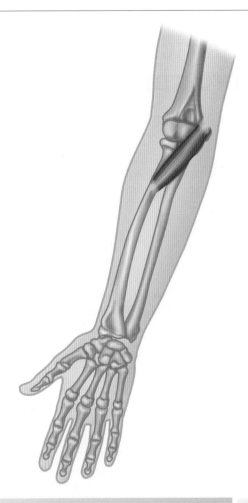

Latin, *pronare*, to bend forward; *teres*, rounded, finely shaped.

Part of the superficial layer of the anterior forearm, which includes flexor carpi radialis, palmaris longus, and flexor carpi ulnaris.

Origin
Humeral head: Lower third of medial supracondylar ridge and the common flexor origin on the anterior aspect of the medial epicondyle of humerus.
Ulnar head: Medial border of the coronoid process of the ulna.

Insertion
Mid-lateral surface of radius (pronator tuberosity).

Action
Pronates forearm. Assists flexion of elbow joint.

Nerve
Median nerve, C6, C7.

Basic functional movement
Example: Pouring liquid from a container. Turning a doorknob.

Movements that may injure this muscle
Repetitive twisting of a heavy or resisting object.

Asanas that heavily use this muscle
Matsyasana. Garudasana (Level I—palms facing out). Reverse Table or *Purvottanasana* with fingers toward hips. *Virabhadrasana II. Viparita Virabhadrasana* (Reverse Warrior, bottom arm).

PRONATOR QUADRATUS

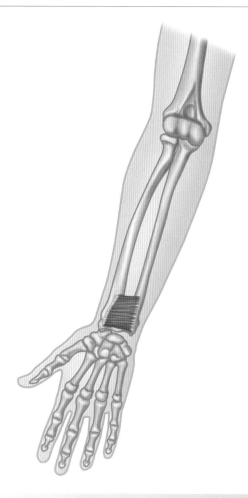

Latin, *pronare*, to bend forward; *quadratus*, squared.

Part of the deep layer of the anterior forearm, which includes flexor digitorum profundus and flexor pollicis longus.

Origin
Distal quarter of anterior surface of shaft of ulna.

Insertion
Lateral side of distal quarter of anterior surface of shaft of radius.

Action
Pronates forearm and hand. Helps hold radius and ulna together, reducing stress on the inferior radioulnar joint.

Nerve
Anterior interosseous branch of median nerve, C7, C8, T1.

Basic functional movement
Turning hand downward as in pouring a substance out of the hand.

Movements that may injure this muscle
Repetitive twisting of a heavy or resisting object.

Asanas that heavily use this muscle
See "Pronator Teres."

Matsyasana (Fish Pose) Level I

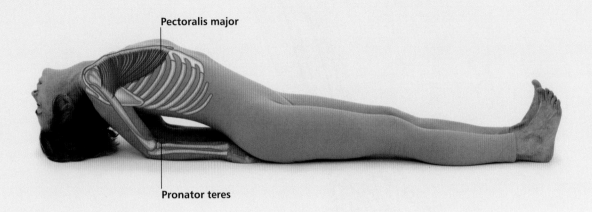

Pectoralis major

Pronator teres

Fish Pose is shown as a strong asana for forearm pronation and wrist/hand extension as they support the upper body, even though the asana action is mainly thoracic hyperextension.

matsya = fish; (mott-see-AHS-anna)

Awareness: Breath, strength, stretch, chest and belly expansion, stimulation of organs and upper chakras.

Action and Alignment: Spine extension to hyperextension, shoulder extension, shoulder girdle adduction, elbow flexion, radioulnar pronation, wrist and hand extension, hip and knee extension, ankle dorsiflexion. The heart is higher than the head, with the lower body extended.

Technique: Lie down in a supine position, with the arms extended under and toward the tailbone; the hands can act as a "pillow" for the sacrum. Root the pelvis into the ground as the rib cage lifts and expands. The elbows will bend naturally as the forearms support the lift of the torso. The head rests back on the floor, pillow, or block.

Helpful Hints: *Note that care must be taken in any inversion of the head if blood pressure has not been checked or if there are retinal eye conditions.* Use a block under the center of the thoracic spine for support, to make the posture more restorative. Close the eyes and relax. Do this posture toward the end of class. It is a good counter pose for inversion balances, such as Headstand and Shoulder Stand.

Counter Pose: *Savasana* (see Appendix 1).

Neutral *Garudasana* (Eagle Pose) See asana explanation under "Supinator." This posture demonstrates the location of the anterior forearm muscles.

SUPINATOR

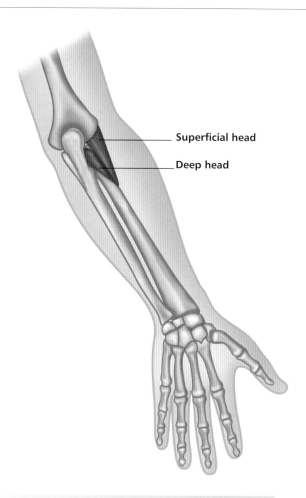

Superficial head

Deep head

Latin, *supinus*, lying on the back.

Part of the deep group of muscles of the posterior forearm. The supinator is almost entirely concealed by the superficial muscles.

Origin
Lower lateral end of humerus (lateral epicondyle) and upper lateral end of ulna and associated ligaments.

Insertion
Dorsal and lateral surfaces of upper third of radius.

Action
Supinates forearm.

Nerve
Deep radial nerve (C5, C6, C7).

Basic functional movement
Example: Turning a door handle or screwdriver.

Remember, supination is also the primary anatomical position. The biceps brachii and the brachioradialis can also aid this action, working synergistically with the supinator muscle—the biceps brachii when the elbow is also flexed, and the brachioradialis when returning from extreme pronation.

Movements that may injure this muscle
Excessive backhand in racket sports. Repetitive twisting of a heavy or resisting object.

Asanas that heavily use this muscle
Full *Garudasana* (Level II). Reverse Table or *Purvottanasana* with fingers away from hips. *Viparita Virabhadrasana* (Reverse Warrior, top arm).

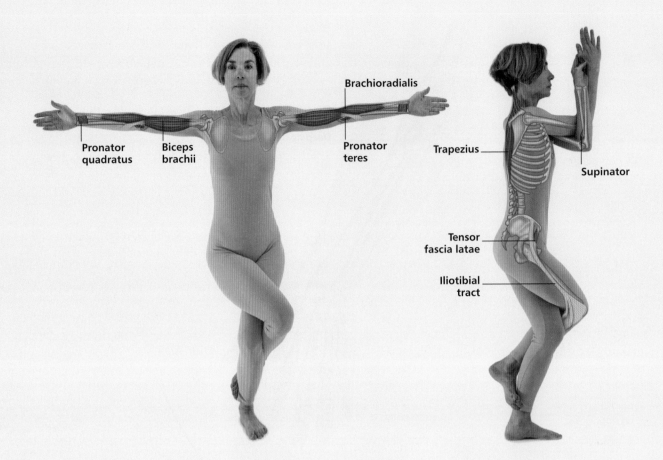

Pronator quadratus
Biceps brachii
Brachioradialis
Pronator teres
Trapezius
Supinator
Tensor fascia latae
Iliotibial tract

Garuda = eagle deity in Indian mythology; (gah-roo-DAHS-anna)

Awareness: Breath, strength, stretch, balance, core stabilization, *drishti*, power, concentration.

Action and Alignment: Spine extension, shoulder horizontal adduction, shoulder girdle protraction (abduction), elbow flexion, radioulnar supination, hip flexion and adduction, knee flexion, ankle dorsiflexion. Upper body is as straight as possible from hips to head.

Technique: Arms—From *Tadasana*, reach the arms out to the sides, then cross in front at the elbows, separating the shoulder blades. Bend the elbows, turning the palms toward one another. Legs—Balance on one leg with the knee slightly bent. Wrap the other leg around, crossing the thighs and creating a "hug" of the legs, with the front foot placed behind the supporting leg. Eagle Pose can be done toward the end of a standing pose sequence.

Helpful Hints: This posture is unique because both shoulders and hips are adducting (frontal plane). As a "chair" position becomes possible, the pelvic floor must be lifted and the core engaged. The tailbone is dropped as the abdominals lift. The gaze is strong and forward. One can place the toes of the front leg on the floor to the outside of the standing foot for support.

Counter Pose: *Tadasana*.

Wrist Joint and Hand

Structure

An important joint in yoga postures supported by the hands, the wrist is termed the "radial carpal joint." This is where the radius and ulna join the carpals, specifically the proximal row, comprising the scaphoid, lunate, triquetrum, and pisiform bones.

The distal row of the carpals, comprising the trapezium, trapezoid, capitate, and hamate, meets the five metacarpals, which articulate with the distal phalanges. Each finger has three phalanges, whereas the thumb has only two. This completes the full hand.

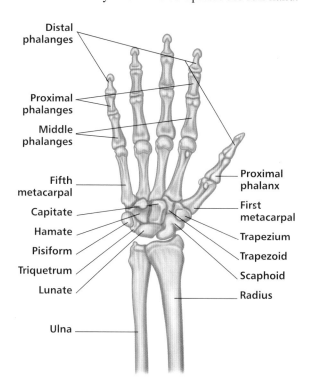

Actions

The wrist is a condyloid joint; therefore, it can do flexion, extension, abduction, and adduction. The combination of these four actions is called "circumduction." When the hand is used as support in yoga postures, the wrist is usually in a hyperextended position. This is a nice counterpoint to a more normal state of the wrist, which is flexion.

The carpometacarpal and metacarpophalangeal joints are also condyloid joints. The interphalangeal joints are hinge joints, where flexion and extension of the fingers occurs.

The thumb is considered a saddle joint. Besides flexion, extension, abduction, and adduction, the action of "opposition" takes place, allowing the thumb to touch each finger separately. Without this action people would not have evolved to this technological age. The specialization of the human hand has enabled us to build fires, make tools, and shape the world. The action of opposition sets humans apart from other primates.

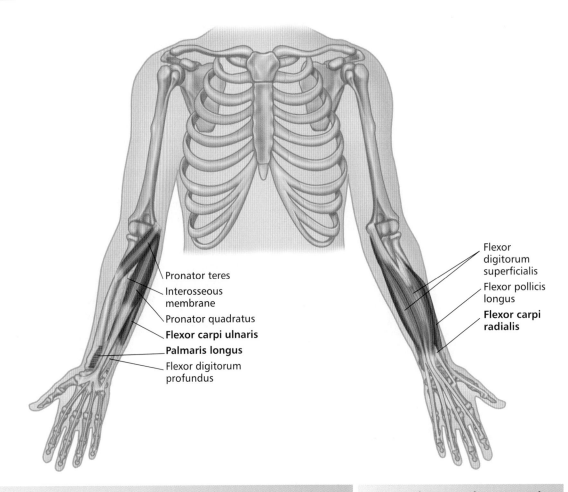

Pronator teres
Interosseous membrane
Pronator quadratus
Flexor carpi ulnaris
Palmaris longus
Flexor digitorum profundus

Flexor digitorum superficialis
Flexor pollicis longus
Flexor carpi radialis

Latin, *flectere*, to bend.

Wrist flexors include flexor carpi radialis, palmaris longus, and flexor carpi ulnaris.

Origin
Common flexor origin on the anterior aspect of the medial epicondyle of humerus (i.e., lower medial end of humerus).

Insertion
Carpals, metacarpals, and phalanges.

Action
Flex the wrist (flexor carpi radialis also abducts the wrist; flexor carpi ulnaris also adducts the wrist).

Nerve
Flexor carpi radialis: Median nerve, C6, C7, C8.
Palmaris longus: Median nerve, C6, C7, C8, T1.
Flexor carpi ulnaris: Ulnar nerve, C7, C8, T1.

Basic functional movement
Example: Pulling a rope in toward you. Wielding an axe or hammer.

Common problems when muscles are chronically tight/shortened/overused
Golfer's elbow (overuse tendonitis of common flexor origin). Carpal tunnel syndrome.

Movements that may injure these muscles
Breaking a fall with the hand.

Asanas that use these muscles
Strengthening: Mudras (hand positions) where forearms are supinated. Circling a clenched fist.
Stretching: Hand Balances. Table Position. *Anjali Mudra* (Prayer Position) and *Pashchima Namaskara* (*Anjali Mudra* Prayer Position behind the back).

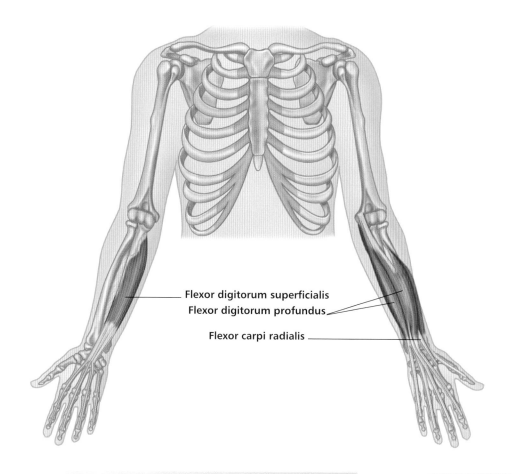

Flexor digitorum superficialis
Flexor digitorum profundus
Flexor carpi radialis

Latin, *flectere*, to bend.

Finger flexors include flexor digitorum superficialis and flexor digitorum profundus.

Origin
Superficialis: Common flexor tendon on medial epicondyle of humerus. Coronoid process of ulna. Anterior border of radius.
Profundus: Medial and anterior surfaces of the ulna.

Insertion
Superficialis: Sides of the middle phalanges of the four fingers.
Profundus: Base of distal phalanges.

Action
Superficialis: Flexes the middle phalanges of each finger. Can help flex the wrist.
Profundus: Flexes distal phalanges (the only muscle able to do so).

Nerve
Superficialis: Median nerve, C7, C8, T1.
Profundus: Medial half of muscle, ulnar nerve, C7, C8, T1; lateral half of muscle, median nerve, C7, C8, T1; sometimes the ulnar nerve supplies the whole muscle.

Basic functional movement
"Hook grip," as in carrying a briefcase. "Power grip," as in turning a tap. Typing. Playing the piano and some stringed instruments.

Common problems when muscles are chronically tight/shortened/overused
Golfer's elbow (overuse tendonitis of common flexor origin). Carpal tunnel syndrome.

Movements or injuries that may damage these muscles
Breaking a fall with the hand.

Asanas that use these muscles
See "Wrist Flexors."

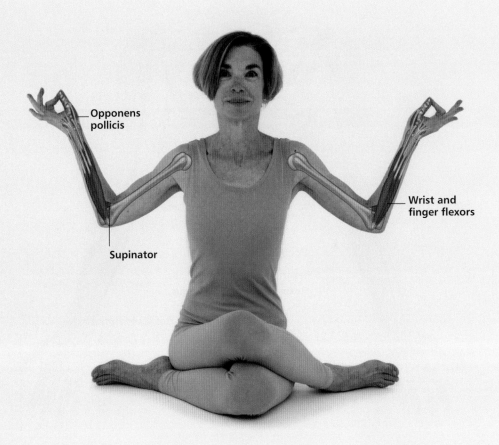

Opponens pollicis

Wrist and finger flexors

Supinator

jnana = knowledge, wisdom; *mudra* = seal, gesture; (jan-ah-mooh-drah)

Awareness: Mind/body connection, energy flow, mental clarity, communication, healing, restorative, centering, peaceful.

Action and Alignment: Spinal extension, hip flexion depending on position, wrist and finger flexion, thumb opposition. Open body for reception.

Technique: In a sitting position, the thumb and index finger touch to create a "seal" and charge of energy.

Helpful Hints: This can be done in any meditation position and incorporated in pranayamas. The index finger relates to Jupiter, the thumb to the ego. It can be performed at any time during class, specifically when awareness needs to be drawn inward. The hand position can be included in many asanas.

Counter Pose: *Savasana* (see Appendix 1).

WRIST EXTENSORS

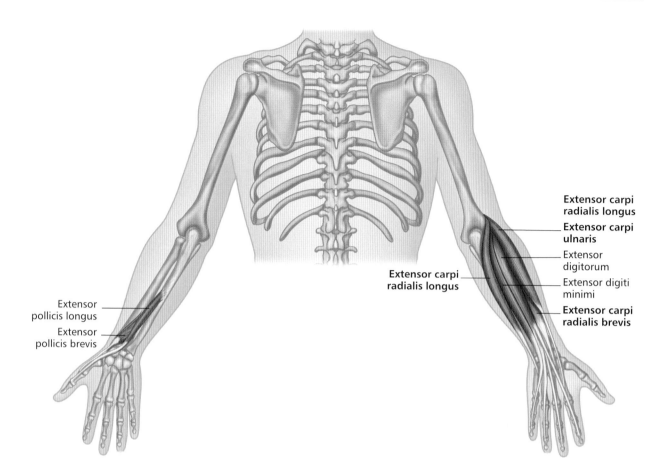

Extensor carpi
radialis longus

Extensor carpi
ulnaris

Extensor
digitorum

Extensor digiti
minimi

Extensor carpi
radialis brevis

Extensor carpi
radialis longus

Extensor
pollicis longus

Extensor
pollicis brevis

Latin, *extendere*, to extend.

Wrist extensors include extensor carpi radialis longus, extensor carpi radialis brevis, and extensor carpi ulnaris.

Origin
Common extensor tendon from lateral epicondyle of humerus (i.e., lower lateral end of humerus).

Insertion
Dorsal surface of metacarpal bones.

Action
Extend the wrist (extensor carpi radialis longus and brevis also abduct the wrist; extensor carpi ulnaris also adducts the wrist).

Nerve
Extensor carpi radialis longus and brevis: Radial nerve, C5, C6, C7, C8.
Extensor carpi ulnaris: Deep radial (posterior interosseous) nerve, C6, C7, C8.

Basic functional movement
Example: Kneading dough. Typing. Cleaning windows.

Common problems when muscles are chronically tight/ shortened/overused
Tennis elbow (overuse tendonitis of common origin on lateral epicondyle of humerus).

Movements that may injure these muscles
Breaking a fall with the hand.

Asanas that heavily use these muscles
Strengthening: Hand balances such as *Adho Mukha Vrksasana* (Handstand). All Plank positions. *Adho* and *Urdhva Mukha Svanasana*.
Stretching: Bring fingers toward inside of wrist (making a fist) and flex the wrist. Clasp hands and circle wrists.

FINGER EXTENSORS (EXTENSOR DIGITORUM)

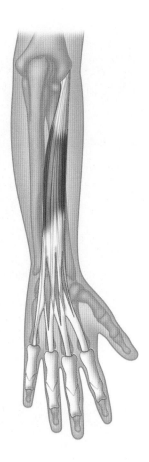

Latin, *extendere*, to extend.

Origin
Common extensor tendon from lateral epicondyle of humerus (i.e., lower lateral end of humerus).

Insertion
Dorsal surfaces of all the phalanges of the four fingers.

Action
Extend the fingers. Assist abduction (divergence) of fingers away from the middle finger.

Nerve
Deep radial (posterior interosseous) nerve, C6, C7, C8.

Basic functional movement
Letting go of objects held in the hand.

Movements that may injure these muscles
Breaking a fall with the hand.

Asanas that heavily use these muscles
See "Wrist Extensors."

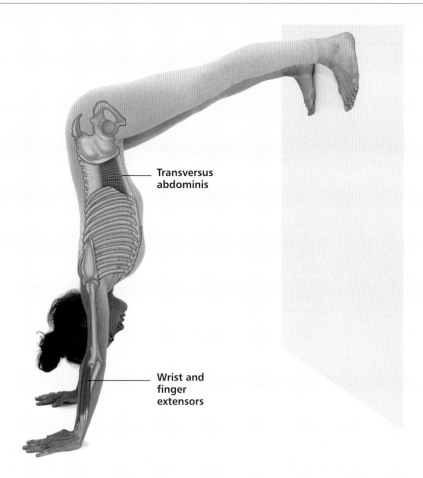

Transversus abdominis

Wrist and finger extensors

adho = downward; *mukha* = face; *vrksasana* = tree; (ahd-hoh moo-kah vrik-SHAHS-anna)

Awareness: Breath, strength, stabilization, core, support, balance, invigoration, determination, calming.

Action and Alignment: Spine extension, shoulder flexion, shoulder girdle stabilization, elbow/wrist/finger extension, hip and knee extension, ankle dorsiflexion or plantar flexion. Torso is neutral and body is aligned as in *Tadasana*, only inverted.

Technique: The asana above is a Level I position because of hip flexion with feet against the wall. (A full handstand is a Level II asana because the arms are supporting the entire weight of the body.) To begin, stand a leg's length away from a blank wall, facing away. Forward bend (*Uttanasana*) to place the hands on the floor, then place the heels against the bottom of the wall in Down Dog position. Take a few breaths here, as this is a great warm-up for the arms and the entire body.

Move the shoulders over the wrists and begin to walk up the wall, one leg at a time, until an inverted "L" position is reached. Hold for up to one minute; the core must work as hard as the arms to balance the posture.

Helpful Hints: *Note that care must be taken in any inversion of the head if blood pressure has not been checked or if there are retinal eye conditions.* It is best to perform this asana using a wall, as it is an extreme strength exercise for the shoulders and arms; there can also be a fear of falling. Once the above technique has been performed, the individual is ready to face the wall and kick up into the handstand. Another person standing to the side can aid the practitioner and help with alignment. This asana is best done toward the end of class, before returning to the floor.

Counter Pose: *Matsyasana* (see above, under "Pronator Quadratus"); *Setu Bandhasana*, *Balasana* (see Chapter 8).

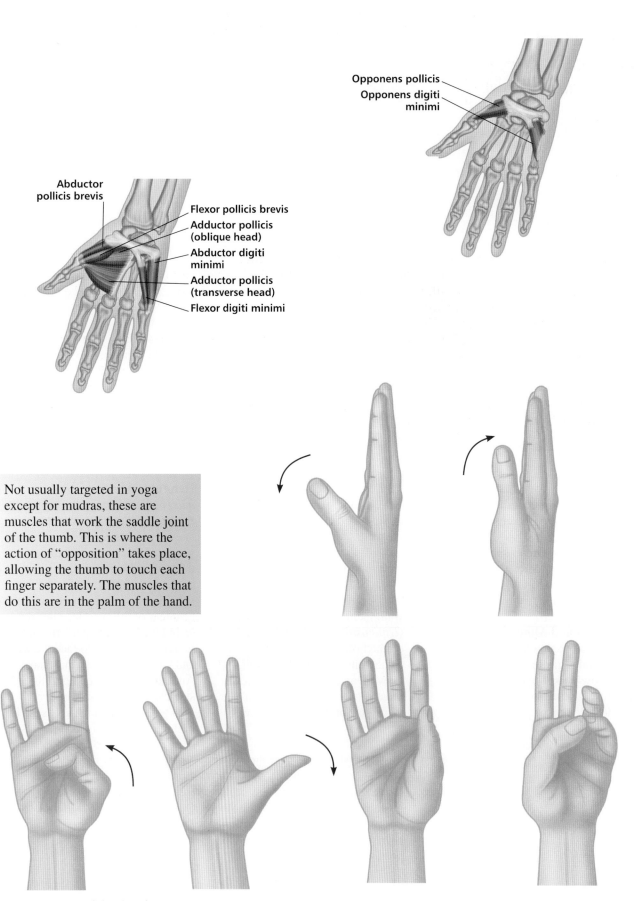

Opponens pollicis
Opponens digiti minimi

Abductor pollicis brevis

Flexor pollicis brevis
Adductor pollicis (oblique head)
Abductor digiti minimi
Adductor pollicis (transverse head)
Flexor digiti minimi

Not usually targeted in yoga except for mudras, these are muscles that work the saddle joint of the thumb. This is where the action of "opposition" takes place, allowing the thumb to touch each finger separately. The muscles that do this are in the palm of the hand.

Opposition of the thumb.

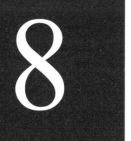

Muscles of the Hip

Hip Joint

The iliofemoral joint, better known as the "hip joint," is the largest ball-and-socket joint in the body and is extremely active in yoga in different ways. It is dominant in standing asanas, whether on one leg or two, and also in backbends as the hip extends along with the spine. The joint is always in a flexed position in forward bends. In sitting postures, such as Lotus, the hips are flexed and outwardly rotated, although the muscles are not in a strongly contracted state. Prone positions, such as Cobra and Bow Pose, stretch the hip flexors and strengthen the extensors, while supine postures can vary greatly. Arm balances also incorporate the hip joint.

Structure

The "ilio" part of this joint's name refers to the iliac bone, a portion of the pelvis which houses the acetabulum of the pelvis (the socket). This cavity articulates with the head of the femur (the ball) to form the joint. In architectural terms, the pelvis is the keystone and the two femurs are the supporting members of an arch-like structure. This makes the hip joint stable and balanced, with excellent structural integrity.

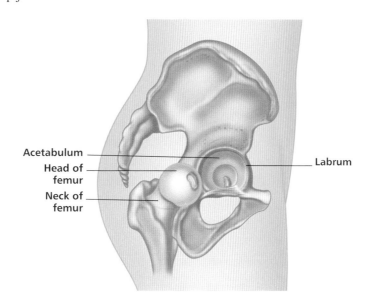

Acetabulum

Head of femur

Neck of femur

Labrum

Connective Tissue

There are three large ligaments that should be noted. The **iliofemoral**, or Y **ligament**, supports the joint anteriorly and limits hip extension and outward rotation. One should consider this while stretching, as an overstretched ligament does not necessarily return to its original length and can make the joint unstable. This is true at any joint and happens often in yoga as students try to go beyond the limits of their body. The **ischiofemoral ligament** originates behind the rim of the socket and crosses the joint to the femur, while the **pubofemoral ligament** extends from the pubis to the fibers of the Y ligament. All work to stabilize and hold the joint together, with other smaller ligaments located around the hip, lumbar, and sacral joints. The **labrum** of the acetabulum is a ring of tissue around the rim of the socket that cushions and stabilizes the joint. It is mentioned here because it is possible to aggravate and even tear this tissue, causing pain around the joint. Structural problems, acute injury, or misuse can lead to this condition, and certain yoga postures can be used to help it.

Actions

Muscles on the front of the thigh flex the hip, the outside (lateral) thigh muscles abduct, the back thigh muscles extend, and the inside (medial) thigh muscles adduct. Most of these muscles also perform inward or outward rotation, the final two actions of the hip. There is a group of six deeper hip rotators that fine-tune outward rotary movements and stabilize the sacral area. Another important component of the lateral thigh is the iliotibial band (ITB), which supports knee stabilization; it comprises the gluteus maximus, tensor fasciae latae, and fascia extending from the pelvis past the knee.

Muscles

The muscles that work the hip pass from the pelvis to the femur, some even going past the knee joint, making these biarticulate. All the larger muscles actually shape the thigh, and most perform more than one action at the hip.

Yoga is a perfect example of balancing strengthening and stretching at the hip joint in all three planes. In Warrior poses the front-leg hip flexors are strengthening as the back-leg flexors are lengthening. In Tree Pose the standing leg is strengthening as the free leg is both strengthening and stretching, depending on the muscle. All of this is described in the muscle and asana illustrations that follow.

In this chapter the muscle information is grouped as flexors, extensors, etc., and an asana will follow each group: one that strengthens, and one that stretches. Of course, there are many asanas that can be included in these areas; some are noted under "Asanas that heavily use this muscle".

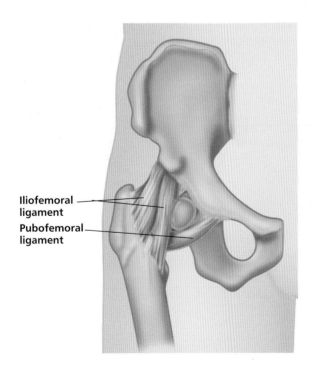

Iliofemoral ligament
Pubofemoral ligament

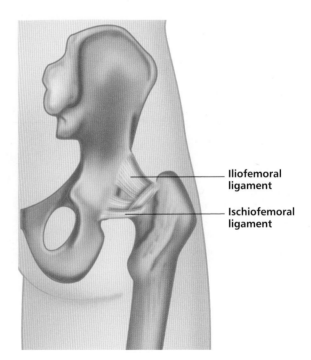

Iliofemoral ligament

Ischiofemoral ligament

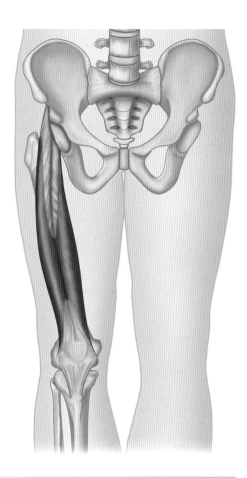

Latin, *rectus*, straight; *femoris*, of the thigh.

Rectus femoris is part of the quadriceps muscle group, which also includes vastus lateralis, vastus medialis, and vastus intermedius (the vasti muscles do not work the hip, only the knee). It has two heads of origin: the reflected head is in the line of pull of the muscle in four-footed animals, whereas the straight head seems to have developed in humans as a result of our upright posture. It is a spindle-shaped, bipennate muscle, which at the hip joint performs only one action—flexion.

Origin
Straight head (anterior head): Anterior inferior iliac spine. Reflected head (posterior head): Groove above acetabulum (on ilium).

Insertion
Patella, then via patellar ligament/quadriceps tendon to tuberosity of tibia.

Action
Extends the knee joint (Chapter 9) and flexes the hip joint (particularly in combination, as in kicking a ball). Prevents flexion at the knee joint as the heel strikes the ground during walking.

Nerve
Femoral nerve, L2, L3, L4.

Basic functional movement
Examples: Walking up stairs. Cycling.

Movements that may injure this muscle
Jumping, landing incorrectly. Sitting too much will weaken it.

Asanas that heavily use this muscle
Most standing postures.
Strengthening: *Utthita Hasta Padangusthasana*. The front leg in *Virabhadrasanas I, II, III*. *Vrksasana*. *Navasana*.
Stretching: *Dhanurasana*. Back leg in *Virabhadrasanas I, II, III*. *Anjaneyasana*. Lunge. Both legs in backbending.

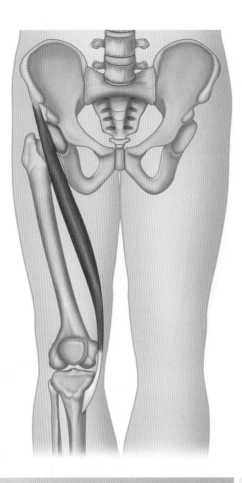

Latin, *sartor*, tailor.

Sartorius is the longest strap muscle in the body. The medial border of the upper third of this muscle forms the lateral boundary of the "femoral triangle" (adductor longus forms the medial boundary, and the inguinal ligament forms the superior boundary). The action of sartorius is to put the lower limbs in the seated cross-legged position of the tailor (hence its name from the Latin), which is also a common meditation and yoga posture.

Origin
Anterior superior iliac spine and the area immediately below it.

Insertion
Upper part of medial surface of tibia, near anterior border.

Action
Flexes the hip joint (helping to bring the leg forward in walking or running). Laterally rotates and abducts the hip joint. Flexes the knee joint. Assists in medial rotation of the tibia on the femur after flexion. Saying that it places the heel on the knee of the opposite limb may summarize these actions (the beginning of a good stretch for the ITB and piriformis).

Nerve
Two branches from the femoral nerve, L2, L3, L4.

Basic functional movement
Example: Sitting cross-legged.

Movements that may injure this muscle
Kicking a heavy ball. Sitting too much will weaken it.

Asanas that heavily use this muscle
(See "Rectus Femoris.") Also: *Sukhasana*, *Padmasana* sitting positions.
Stretching: *Supta Virasana* (Reclined Hero Pose).

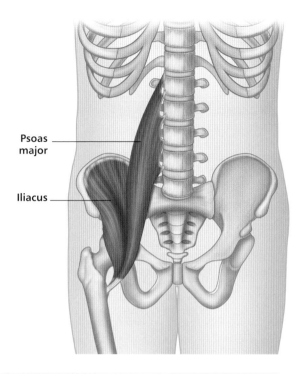

Psoas major

Iliacus

Greek, *psoa*, muscle of the loin. **Latin**, *major*, larger; *iliacus*, pertaining to the loin.

The psoas major and iliacus are considered part of the posterior abdominal wall because of their position and cushioning role for the abdominal viscera. However, the main action of these muscles, particularly the iliacus, is flexion of the hip joint; the psoas major is more of a stabilizer because of its position at the lumbar spine as well as the hip (see Chapter 4).

There is a third muscle that is usually placed in this group, the psoas minor, but as it slowly evolves away from the human body, it is not pictured here. See *The Vital Psoas Muscle* (Staugaard-Jones 2012) for more information about this fascinating area.

Origin
Psoas major: Bases of transverse processes of all lumbar vertebrae (L1–L5). Bodies of twelfth thoracic and all lumbar vertebrae (T12–L5). Intervertebral discs above each lumbar vertebra.

Iliacus: Superior two-thirds of iliac fossa. Anterior ligaments of the lumbosacral and sacroiliac joints.

Insertion
Lesser trochanter of femur.

Action
Psoas major: Mostly a stabilizer of the lumbar and hip joints; weak flexor.
Iliacus: Strong flexor of hip joint (flexes and may laterally rotate the thigh, as in kicking a football, along with sartorius).

Nerve
Psoas major: Ventral rami of lumbar nerves, L1, L2, L3, L4.
Iliacus: Femoral nerve, L1, L2, L3, L4.

Basic functional movement
Example: Going up a step or walking up an incline.

Common problems when muscles are chronically tight/shortened
Lower back pain due to increase in lumbar curve (lordosis). Bilateral contracture of this muscle will increase lumbar lordosis.

Asanas that heavily use this muscle
See asanas under "Rectus Femoris."
Strengthening: *Utthita Hasta Padangusthasana* (Extended Hand-to-Big-Toe Balance).
Stretching: *Setu Bandhasana* (Half Bridge Pose).

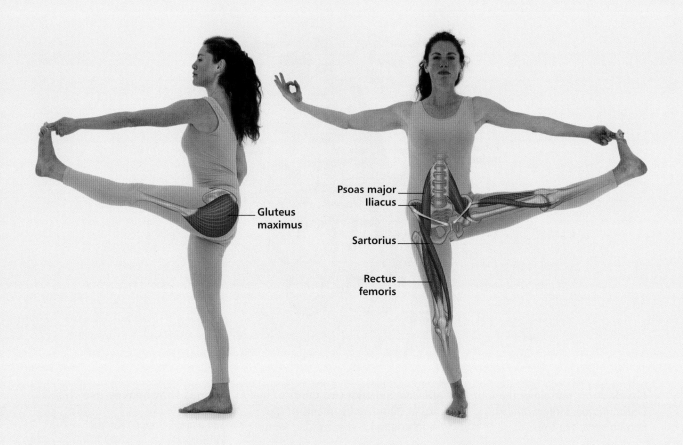

Gluteus maximus

Psoas major
Iliacus

Sartorius

Rectus femoris

utthita = extended; *hasta* = hand; *pada* = foot; *angusta* = big toe; (oo-TE-ta ha-stah pad-ahn-goos-TAHS-anna)

Awareness: Breath, strength, stretch, balance, core, concentration, *drishti*.

Action and Alignment: Spine extension, shoulder stabilization, hip flexion to outward rotation, knee extension, ankle dorsiflexion. Body stays aligned from the head to the toe on the standing side.

Technique: From *Tadasana*, shift the weight over to one foot as the other leg lifts to bend the knee to the chest. Take hold of the big toe of the free leg and begin to extend the leg to the front. If possible, let go of the toe and hold the leg parallel to the ground, with the spine extended straight up. It is best to do this pose once the hip flexors and extensors have been warmed up.

Helpful Hints: In this one-leg balance, it is important not to lean back as the leg extends to the front. Use a wall and/or strap for more support. Keep the pelvis centered. For more of a challenge, extend the leg out the side, looking in the opposite direction to the raised leg (this is called *Supta Padangusthasana*). One can also hold onto the bent knee for a Level I exercise. The gluteus maximus is shown in the left hand photograph as as lengthening muscle.

Counter Pose: *Tadasana*.

Setu Bandhasana (Half Bridge Pose) Level I (Hip Flexor Stretch)

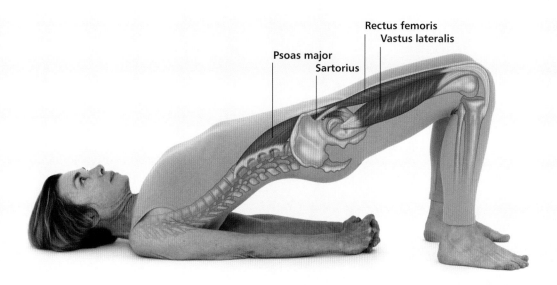

Psoas major
Sartorius
Rectus femoris
Vastus lateralis

setu = bridge; *bandha* = lock; (Set-too bahn-DAHS-anna)

Awareness: Breath, stretch, strength, stimulation, circulation, calming, therapeutic.

Action and Alignment: Spine hyperextension, shoulder stabilization, hip extension, knee flexion. Shoulders are firm on the floor, and knees are over the feet.

Technique: From a supine position, bend the knees and position the feet flat on the floor, hip-width apart. Place the arms along the sides of the hips with palms facing down, and reach the fingers toward the heels. Push the pelvis up off the ground, ideally in line with the knees. If the hips are high enough, clasp the hands underneath and bring the shoulder blades closer together.

Helpful Hints: To make this more comfortable and restorative, allow the sacrum to rest on a block. Either way, it is a great hip opener and can be done at any time during class when this is needed.

Counter Pose: *Savasana* (see Appendix 1).

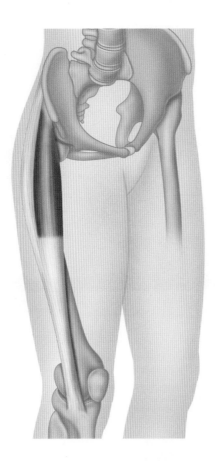

Latin, *tendere*, to stretch, pull; *fasciae*, of the band; *latae*, broad.

This muscle lies anterior to gluteus maximus, on the lateral side of the hip.

Origin
Anterior part of outer lip of iliac crest and outer surface of anterior superior iliac spine.

Insertion
Joins iliotibial tract just below level of greater trochanter.

Action
Flexes, abducts, and medially rotates the hip joint. Tenses the fascia lata, thus stabilizing the knee. Redirects the rotational forces produced by the gluteus maximus.

Nerve
Superior gluteal nerve, L4, L5, S1.

Basic functional movement
Example: Walking.

Movements that may injure this muscle
Excessive running, hiking, cycling, squatting.

Asanas that heavily use this muscle
Strengthening: *Parighasana* (Gate Pose). *Prasarita Padottanasana* (Wide-leg Forward Bend). Most standing asanas, as abductors stabilize.
Stretching: *Supta Matsyendrasana* (Supine Spinal Twist). *Eka Pada Kapotasana* (Pigeon Pose, front leg).

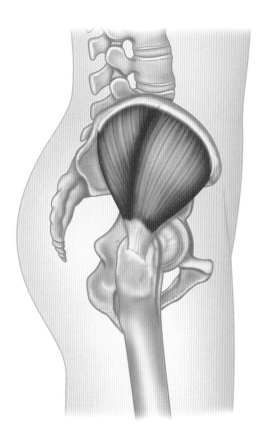

Greek, *gloutos*, buttock. **Latin**, *medius*, middle.

This muscle is mostly deep to, and therefore obscured by, gluteus maximus but appears on the surface between gluteus maximus and tensor fasciae latae. During walking, this muscle, along with gluteus minimus, prevents the pelvis from dropping toward the non-weight-bearing leg.

Origin
Outer surface of ilium, inferior to iliac crest, between posterior and anterior gluteal lines.

Insertion
Oblique ridge on lateral surface of greater trochanter of femur.

Action
Abducts the hip joint. Anterior fibers medially rotate and may assist in flexion of the hip joint. Posterior fibers slightly laterally rotate the hip joint.

Nerve
Superior gluteal nerve, L4, L5, S1.

Basic functional movement
Example: Stepping sideways over an object, such as a low fence.

See "Tensor Fasciae Latae" for movements that may injure the gluteus medius, and also for asanas.

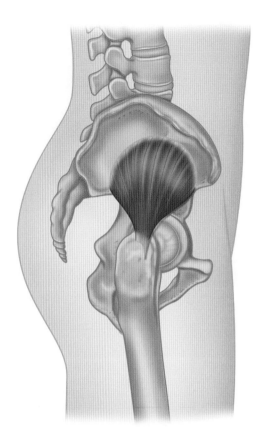

Greek, *gloutos*, buttock. **Latin**, *minimus*, smallest.

This muscle is situated anteroinferior and deep to gluteus medius, whose fibers obscure it.

Origin
Outer surface of ilium, between anterior and inferior gluteal lines.

Insertion
Anterior border of greater trochanter.

Action
Abducts, medially rotates, and may assist in flexion of the hip joint.

Nerve
Superior gluteal nerve, L4, L5, S1.

Basic functional movement
Example: Stepping sideways over an object, such as a low fence.

See "Tensor Fasciae Latae" for movements that may injure the gluteus minimus.

Asanas that heavily use this muscle
Strengthening: *Parighasana* (Crossbar or Gate Pose).
Stretching: *Supta Matsyendrasana* (Reclined or Supine Spinal Twist), or the counter pose, see opposite. See also "Tensor Fasciae Latae" for asanas.

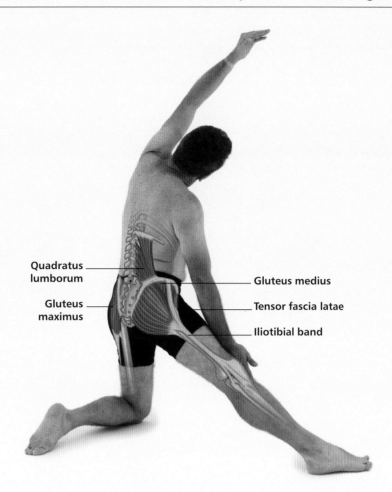

Quadratus lumborum

Gluteus maximus

Gluteus medius

Tensor fascia latae

Iliotibial band

parigha = gate latch; (par-eh-GOSS-anna)

Awareness: Breath, strength, stretch, lateral movement, core, balance.

Action and Alignment: Spine lateral flexion, shoulder girdle rotation, shoulder joint abduction, hip abduction, knee flexion and extension. The body remains in the frontal plane.

Technique: From a kneeling position, extend one leg out to the side, with the knee and toes facing forward. Extend the arms out to the sides, with the pelvis even. Laterally bend the spine up and over toward the straight leg as the opposite arm reaches over the head; press the shoulder down. The back of the bottom hand can rest on the inside calf of the bottom leg. The gaze is forward. For more strength work, lift the torso up and over to the other side, then lift the straight leg; hold and balance.

Helpful Hints: For a variation, outwardly rotate the straight leg. Both sides of the ribs need to lengthen. If one cannot kneel because of a knee injury, this pose can be done on a chair. It is important to include this pose in any class, as it works the body in the frontal plane, whereas many asanas are done in the sagittal plane. Balance is the key. It can be performed at any time during class, preferably when the practitioner is already down on the mat.

Counter Pose: Lift the torso up and over to the other side, then change sides.

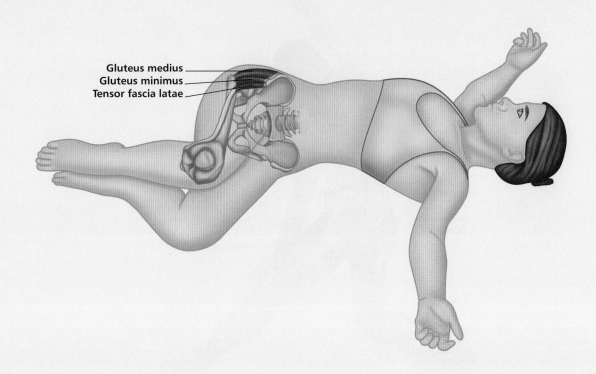

Gluteus medius
Gluteus minimus
Tensor fascia latae

supta = reclined; *Matsyendrasana* = Lord of the Fishes; (Soop-tah MAHT-see-en-DRAHS-anna)

Awareness: Breath, stretch, spinal release, relaxation, digestion, massage of organs.

Action and Alignment: Spine rotation, shoulder joint abduction, hip flexion and adduction, knee flexion. Shoulder blades remain on the ground, with the spine lengthened.

Technique: From a supine position, hug both knees to the chest, then place the arms out to the sides. Allow the legs to rest on the ground to one side. The head can turn to the opposite side for more rotation of the cervical area. It is best to breathe here and rest. To bring the legs back up, exhale to engage the core to help. A variation is to extend one leg up and over to the opposite side for more stretch, or extend the bottom leg.

Helpful Hints: For those with lower back or hip issues, it is advised to rest the knees to the side on a blanket or block so the lower spine does not twist as much. If there is a shoulder problem, do not extend that arm out. This posture is best done at the beginning or end of class, and is a good stretch for the sacroiliac joint as well as the ITB: a combination of the tensor fascia lata, gluteus maximus and a tract of connective tissue that extends past the knee and is often tight.

Counter Pose: *Savasana* (see Appendix 1).

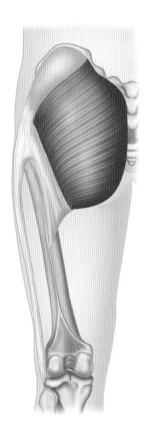

Greek, *gloutos*, buttock. **Latin,** *maximus*, biggest.

The gluteus maximus is the most coarsely fibered and heaviest muscle in the body.

Origin
Outer surface of ilium, behind posterior gluteal line and portion of bone superior and posterior to it. Adjacent posterior surface of sacrum and coccyx. Sacrotuberous ligament. Aponeurosis of erector spinae.

Insertion
Deep fibers of distal portion: Gluteal tuberosity of femur. Remaining fibers: Iliotibial tract of fascia lata.

Action
Upper fibers: Laterally rotate hip joint. May assist in abduction of hip joint.
Lower fibers: Extend and laterally rotate hip joint (forceful extension as in running or rising from sitting). Extend trunk. Assists in adduction of hip joint.
Through its insertion into the iliotibial tract, it helps stabilize the knee in extension.

Nerve
Inferior gluteal nerve, L5, S1, S2.

Basic functional movement
Examples: Walking upstairs. Rising from sitting.

Movements that may injure this muscle
Excessive jumping, running, hiking, cycling, stair climbing, squatting.

Asanas that heavily use this muscle
Strengthening: *Setu Bandhasana. Virabhadrasanas I, II, III* (back leg). Backbends, such as *Bhujangasana, Salabhasana, Ustrasana, Urdhva Dhanurasana* (Full Wheel).
Stretching: *Balasana* (Child's Pose). *Ananda Balasana* (Happy Baby). Supine/Reclined Twists. Forward Bends.

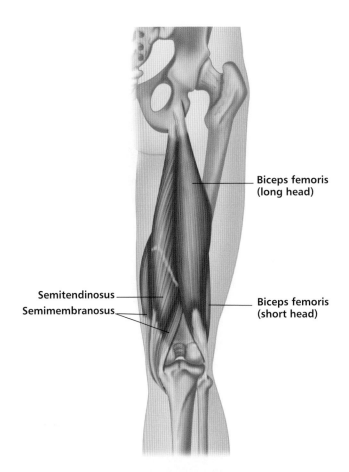

Biceps femoris (long head)

Semitendinosus

Semimembranosus

Biceps femoris (short head)

German, *hamme*, back of leg; **Latin**, *stringere*, to draw together.

The hamstrings consist of three muscles. From medial to lateral these are the semimembranosus, semitendinosus, and biceps femoris.

Origin
Ischial tuberosity (sitting bone). Biceps femoris also originates from the back of the femur.

Insertion
Semimembranosus: Back of medial condyle of tibia (upper inside part of tibia). Semitendinosus: Upper medial surface of shaft of tibia. Biceps femoris: Head (top) of fibula. Lateral condyle of tibia (upper outside part of tibia).

Action
Flex the knee joint. Extend the hip joint. Semimembranosus and semitendinosus also medially rotate (turn in) the lower leg when the knee is flexed. Biceps femoris laterally rotates (turns out) the lower leg when the knee is flexed.

Nerve
Branches of the sciatic nerve, L4, L5, S1, S2, S3.

Basic functional movement
During running, the hamstrings slow down the leg at the end of its forward swing and prevent the trunk from flexing at the hip joint.

Common problems when muscles are chronically tight/ shortened
Lower back pain. Knee pain. Leg-length discrepancies. Restriction of stride length in walking or running.

Movements or injuries that may damage these muscles
Sudden lengthening of the muscle (e.g., forward kicking, splits) without sufficient warm-up.

Asanas that heavily use these muscles
Strengthening: *Dhanurasana* (Bow Pose). See also "Gluteus Maximus."
Stretching: *Balasana* (Child's Pose). Forward Bends with knees straight, such as *Paschimottanasana* and *Adho Mukha Svanasana*. *Halasana* (Plow Pose).

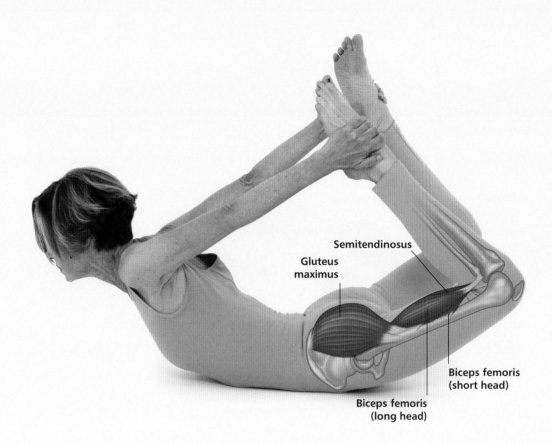

Semitendinosus

Gluteus maximus

Biceps femoris (short head)

Biceps femoris (long head)

dhanu = bow; (don-ur-AHS-anna)

Awareness: Breath, stretch, strength, chest expansion, flexibility, stimulation of organs.

Action and Alignment: Spine hyperextension, shoulder girdle adduction, shoulder joint hyperextension, hip extension, knee flexion to extension, ankle dorsiflexion. The body is arched like a "bow," with shoulders and knees in line with each other.

Technique: Begin in a prone position. For Level I, bend one knee and reach back for the foot with the same hand. Grab the ankle, push the foot into the hand, and lift the thigh as well as the torso. Extend the opposite arm out in front, then repeat on the other side. For Level II, do both legs at the same time and try to keep the knees close to one another. The gaze is forward.

Helpful Hints: It is best to warm up with Level I before advancing to Level II. Use the pressing of the feet into the hands to lift the chest. Breathe deeply. This pose is usually done toward the end of class, when the hips need to open and the spine has been warmed up. Level II is an intense backbend.

Counter Pose: *Makarasana* (see Chapter 6).

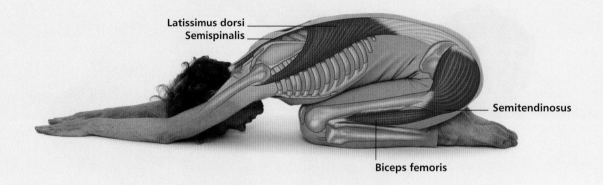

bala = child; (baa-LAHS-anna)

Awareness: Breath, stretch, release, calming, stimulation of organs, relaxation, restorative.

Action and Alignment: Spine flexion, shoulder girdle upward rotation (arms reaching forward), shoulder joint flexion, hip and knee flexion, ankle plantar flexion. Body is in the sagittal plane.

Technique: From a kneeling position, such as *Vajrasana*, forward bend over the thighs (big toes are together, knees separated slightly). Sit toward or on the heels. Reach the arms forward, or place them by the sides of the body. Hold for a minute or more for a deep release.

Helpful Hints: If there is a hip, knee, or ankle problem, place a blanket between the hips and the ankles. One can also lie on a bolster. The head can rest on the hands or a blanket if the neck is compromised. This posture is a great spine lengthener, and can be done at any time when rest is needed.

Counter Pose: *Savasana* (see Appendix 1).

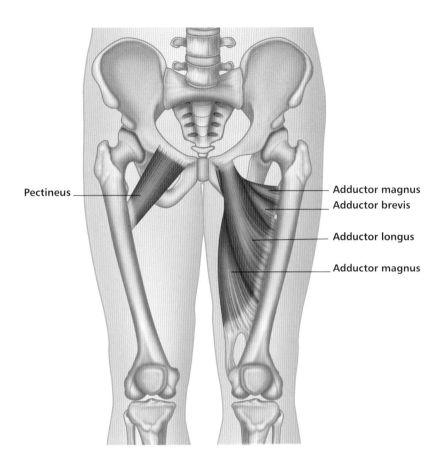

Pectineus

Adductor magnus
Adductor brevis

Adductor longus

Adductor magnus

Latin, *adducere*, to lead to; *magnus*, large; *brevis*, short; *longus*, long.

The adductor magnus is the largest of the adductor muscle group, which also includes adductor brevis and adductor longus. Adductor longus is the most anterior of the three. The lateral border of the upper fibers of adductor longus form the medial border of the femoral triangle (sartorius forms the lateral boundary; the inguinal ligament forms the superior boundary).

Origin
Anterior part of pubic bone (ramus). Adductor magnus also takes its origin from the ischial tuberosity.

Insertion
Entire length of medial side of femur, from the hip to the knee.

Action
Adduct and laterally rotate hip joint.

Nerve
Magnus: Obturator nerve, L2, L3, L4. Sciatic nerve, L4, L5, S1. Brevis and Longus: Obturator nerve, L2, L3, L4.

Basic functional movement
Example: Bringing second leg in or out of a car.

Common problems when muscles are chronically tight/shortened/fatigued
Groin pulls.

Movements or injuries that may damage these muscles
Side splits or high side-kicks without sufficient warm-up.

Asanas that heavily use these muscles
Strengthening: *Parsvottanasana*. All standing asanas using the adductors as stabilizers.
Stretching: *Baddha Konasana. Ananda Balasana* (Happy Baby). *Upavistha Konasana* (Wide-leg Straddle). *Prasarita Padottanasana*.

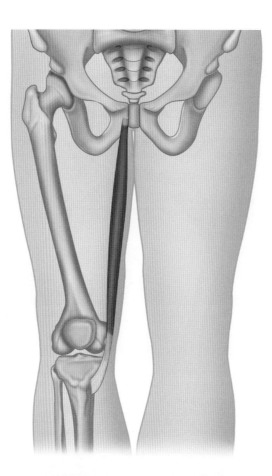

Latin, *gracilis*, slender, delicate.

Gracilis descends down the medial side of the thigh, anterior to semimembranosus.

Origin
Lower half of symphysis pubis and inferior ramus of pubis.

Insertion
Upper part of medial surface of shaft of tibia.

Action
Adducts hip joint. Flexes knee joint. Medially rotates knee joint when flexed.

Nerve
Anterior division of obturator nerve, L2, L3, L4.

Basic functional movement
Example: Sitting with knees pressed together.

Asanas that heavily use this muscle
Strengthening: *Parsvottanasana*. All standing asanas using the adductors as stabilizers.
Stretching: *Baddha Konasana*. *Ananda Balasana* (Happy Baby). *Upavistha Konasana* (Wide-leg Straddle). *Prasarita Padottanasana*.

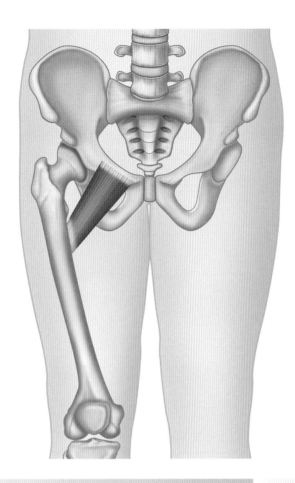

Latin, *pecten*, comb; *pectinatus*, comb shaped.

Pectineus is sandwiched between the psoas major and adductor longus.

Origin
Pecten of pubis, between iliopubic (iliopectineal) eminence and pubic tubercle.

Insertion
Pectineal line, from lesser trochanter to linea aspera of femur.

Action
Adducts the hip joint. Flexes the hip joint.

Nerve
Femoral nerve, L2, L3, L4. Occasionally receives an additional branch from the obturator nerve, L3.

Basic functional movement
Example: Walking along a straight line.

Common problems when muscles are chronically tight/shortened/fatigued
Groin pulls.

Asanas that heavily use this muscle
Strengthening: *Parsvottanasana* (Pyramid Pose). All standing asanas using the adductors as stabilizers.
Stretching: *Baddha Konasana* (Bound Angle Pose). *Supta Konasana* (Reclined Straddle Pose) to *Ananda Balasana* (Happy Baby). *Upavistha Konasana* (Wide-leg Straddle). *Prasarita Padottanasana*.

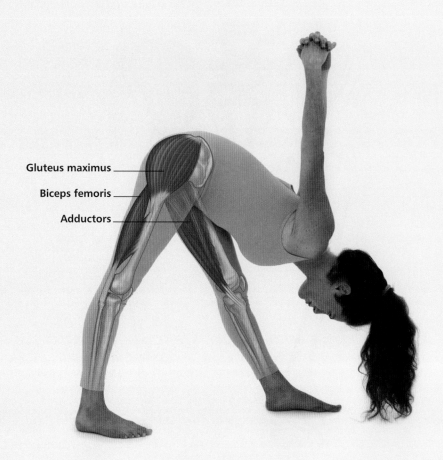

Gluteus maximus

Biceps femoris

Adductors

parsva = side; *ut* = intense; *tan* = stretch, extend; (pars-vo-tahn-AHS-anna)

Awareness: Breath, strength, stretch, core engagement, balance, concentration, stimulation, energizing.

Action and Alignment: Spine extension, shoulder girdle stabilization, shoulder extension, hip flexion, knee extension. Body remains in the sagittal plane, with the feet lined up with one another if possible.

Technique: From *Tadasana*, step back with one leg, placing the foot facing forward with the heel down. Extend the arms and clasp the hands behind the back. Fold the torso forward over the front thigh, staying in line with it. Stop halfway when the torso is extended and parallel to the floor; take a full breath. Continue to fold to the front thigh as the arms are lifted up behind. The hip adductors are working to keep the legs in a parallel position, front to back and underneath the body.

Helpful Hints: Reach for the floor or blocks on either side of the front foot for support. Push the front hip back and the back hip forward to square the hips. Keep the knees extended, but not locked. This is an intense stretch for the backs of the legs and the spine. Engage the core and lift the pelvic floor to support and balance the posture. Do this pose after the body has been warmed up well.

Counter Pose: *Tadasana* with arms raised and a slight backbend (Crescent).

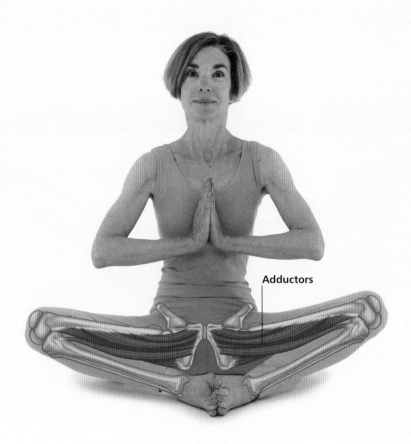

Adductors

baddha = bound; *kona* = angle; (Bah-dah cone-AHS-anna)

Awareness: Breath, stretch, stimulation, circulation, calming, supports lower chakras.

Action and Alignment: Spine extension, shoulder stabilization, hip flexion and outward rotation, knee flexion, ankle dorsiflexion. The mid-ear and the hip are in line.

Technique: In a sitting position, bend the knees and place the soles of the feet together. Extend the spine, sitting on top of the sit bones. Clasp the ankles or toes with the hands. Begin to hinge forward from the hips, keeping the spine straight, for more stretch. Once this is achieved, one can round over the legs.

Helpful Hints: It is most important to keep the spine straight at the beginning, so the feet may have to be pushed out further in front, or one can sit higher on a blanket or block, or against the wall. This is a good posture toward the beginning of class, and can be used in meditation or pranayamas.

Counter Pose: *Bharadvajasana* (see Chapter 4).

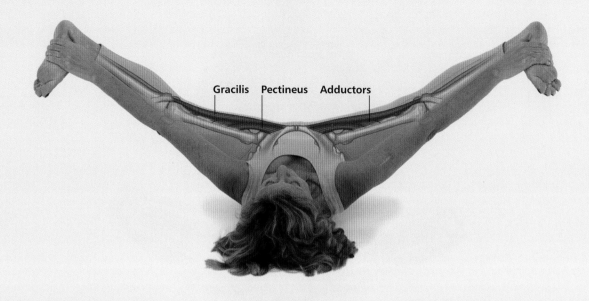

Gracilis   Pectineus   Adductors

supta = reclined; *kona* = angle; (Soop-tah cone-AHS-anna) *ananda* = bliss; *bala* = child; (ah-NAHN-da baa-LAHS-anna)

Awareness: Breath, stretch, stimulation, circulation, stress relief, openness.

Action and Alignment: Spine extension, hip flexion to outward rotation to abduction, knee flexion and extension, ankle dorsiflexion. The ground maintains spinal alignment.

Technique: In a supine position, hug the knees into the chest, then bring the legs to a *Baddha Konasana* position, holding the toes or ankles. Straighten the knees and extend the legs out to a straddle position.

Helpful Hints: Place the hands on the insides or outsides of the thighs for support as the legs extend. Breathe deeply and enjoy. This is a nice hip opener, and can be done toward the end of class, as with Happy Baby (a reclined position in which the knees are bent into the ribs and the feet are held as the thighs flex and separate).

Counter Pose: Happy Baby, then *Savasana* (see Appendix 1).

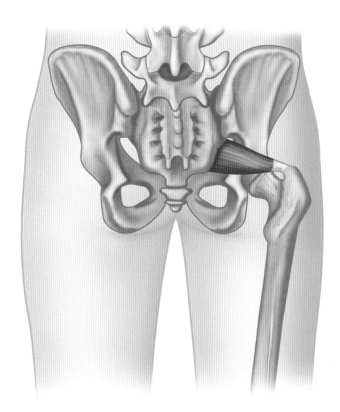

Latin, *pirum*, pear; *forma*, shape.

The largest of the six deep outward rotators of the hip, the piriformis leaves the pelvis by passing through the greater sciatic foramen, posterior to the sciatic nerve, and is thus a culprit in the impingement of this nerve (sciatica).

Origin
Internal surface of sacrum. Sacrotuberous ligament.

Insertion
Superior border of greater trochanter of femur.

Action
Laterally rotates hip joint. Abducts the thigh when hip is flexed. Helps hold head of femur in acetabulum.

Nerve
Ventral rami of lumbar nerve, L5, and sacral nerves, S1, S2.

Basic functional movement
Example: Taking the first leg out of a car. In yoga, outward rotation of the hip, as in sitting meditation postures.

See asana list on the next page.

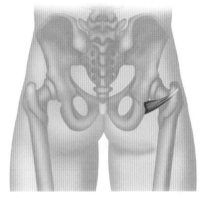

Obturator externus

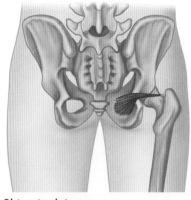

Obturator internus

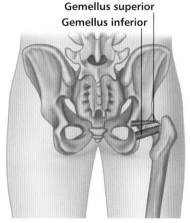

Gemellus superior
Gemellus inferior

Gemelli

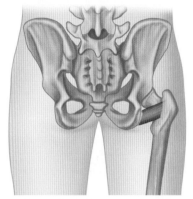

Quadratus femoris

Latin, *obturare*, to obstruct; *gemellus*, twin/double; *quadratus*, squared; *femoris*, of the thigh.

Origin
Obturator externus: Between the margin of the foramen and the attachment of the obturator membrane.
Obturator internus: Inner surface of ischium, pubis, and ilium.
Gemellus superior: Ischial spine (lower posterior area of pelvis).
Gemellus inferior: Just below Origin of gemellus superior.
Quadratus femoris: Lateral edge of ischial tuberosity (sitting bone).

Insertion
Greater trochanter (top) of femur (except quadratus femoris, which inserts just behind and below the others).

Action
Laterally rotates hip joint. Helps hold head of femur in its socket (acetabulum).

Nerve
Obturator internus and gemellus superior: Nerve to obturator internus, L5, S1, S2.
Gemellus inferior and quadratus femoris: Nerve to quadratus femoris, L4, L5, S1, S2.

Basic functional movement
Example: Taking the first leg out of a car.

Common problems when muscles are chronically tight/shortened
Person stands with feet turned out. Sciatic nerve can be impinged by piriformis.

Movements that may injure these muscles
Insufficient warm-up for sideward kicking, breaststroke, ballet.

Asanas that heavily use these muscles
Strengthening: *Ardha Chandrasana* (Half Moon Pose), top leg. *Utkata Konasana* (Goddess Pose). *Padmasana*. *Baddha Konasana*. *Vrksasana* (bent leg). *Janu Sirsasana* (bent leg).
Stretching: *Eka Pada Kapotasana* (Pigeon Pose) variation. *Gomukasana* (legs). *Ardha Matsyendrasana* (Sitting Twist, bent leg). Crossed Leg Stretch.

Note: Hip inward rotation positions will stretch these muscles the most, but the placement of the front leg closer to hip adduction (across the midline) in Pigeon can help lengthen the piriformis, which may release pressure on the sciatic nerve.

Secondary muscles that outwardly rotate the hip are sartorius, gluteus maximus, biceps femoris, and the adductor group.

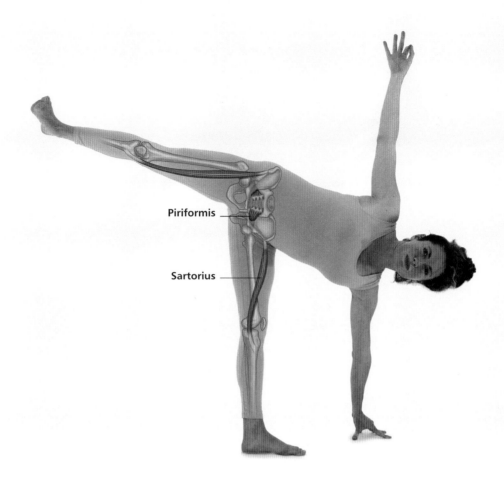

Piriformis

Sartorius

ardha = half; *chandra* = shining moon; (ard-hah chan-DRAHS-anna)

Awareness: Breath, strength, stretch, balance, openness, coordination, *drishti*.

Action and Alignment: Spine extension, shoulder girdle stabilization, shoulder joint abduction, hip flexion and outward rotation, knee extension, ankle dorsiflexion. The body remains in a flat plane, with the shoulders in line with each other (stacked).

Technique: From *Trikonasana*, bend the front knee, then extend as the back leg lifts to a high, outwardly rotated position. The bottom arm reaches to the floor or a block, while the top arm lifts to the sky.

Helpful Hints: This posture is best done against a wall, as the practitioner can experience the back of their body with a flat support behind them, which brings them into a neutral plane. Level II is when no support is used. The pose can be done in the second half of class, when warm-ups for the hips have already been performed.

Counter Pose: *Tadasana*, then do *Ardha Chandrasana* on the other side.

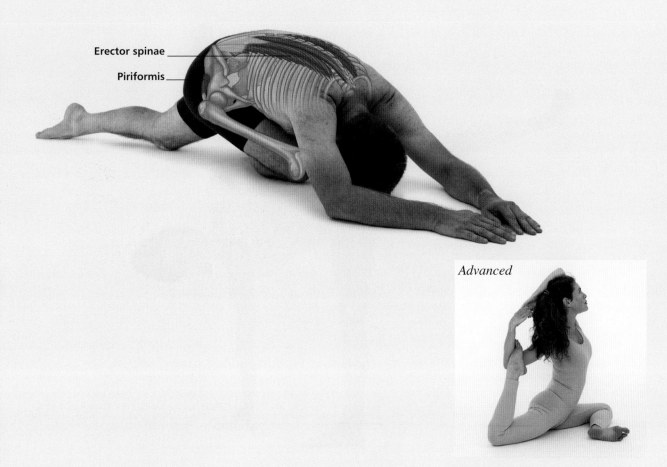

Erector spinae

Piriformis

Advanced

eka = one; *pada* = foot, leg; *raja* = king; *kapota* = pigeon/dove; (eh-kah pah-dah rah-jah-cop-poh-TAHS-anna)

Awareness: Breath, stretch, strength, balance, core, shoulder, chest, and hip opener, backbend (when upright), stimulation of organs.

Action and Alignment: Spine extension to hyperextension (upright), shoulder girdle and core stabilization, shoulder joint flexion (hyperextension if doing advanced version), hip flexion/rotation (front leg), hip extension (back leg), knee flexion and extension. The mid-ear to the hip is in alignment, whether upright or reclined.

Technique: From Table, Down Dog, or Plank, slide one knee forward in between the hands as the back leg stretches behind. The weight of the body will rest into the hips, which intensifies the stretch. Lift the pelvic floor and core to help reduce the pressure, or use a support. From this upright position, reach the arms forward on the ground to a reclined position (shown).

This posture is commonly known as a piriformis stretch in the front leg, but it depends on the position. There is more stretch if the front knee begins to cross the midline toward the opposite side. Another stretch is *Adho Muka Virasana* (Downward Facing Hero Pose), sitting with the legs inwardly rotated (knees bent) then folding forward (the frontal version of page 157). If the knees cannot bend at this angle, straighten them but still inwardly rotate the thighs as the hips flex.

Helpful Hints: This is a difficult posture when the hips are tight, a condition that affects many people. Use a blanket or block for support under the front hip if needed. Any lift of the hips off the floor will ease the posture, as long as the arms are supportive as well. Keep an eye on the integrity of the knees: the front one will be in a deeply bent position, and the back one may need a soft support. The advanced version is also shown, just for fun. Pigeon is best done from the middle toward the end of class, when the hips have already been warmed up.

Counter Pose: *Makarasana* (Crocodile).

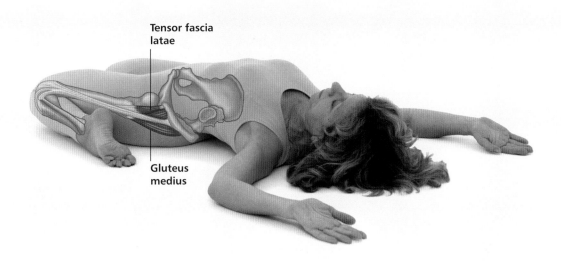

supta = reclining; *vira* = hero;
(Soop-tah veer-AHS-anna)

Awareness: Breath, anterior
stretch, hip opener, digestion,
relaxation.

Action and Alignment: Spine
extension to hyperextension,
shoulder stabilization, hip
extension and internal rotation,
knee flexion, ankle plantar flexion.
Body is in a reclined straight line.

Technique: From *Virasana*
(similar to *Vajrasana*, Chapter 2,
with the lower legs outside the
thighs), begin to lie back on the
forearms. If this is comfortable,
recline all the way back.

The abdominals, hip flexors,
quadriceps, and ankles will
stretch immensely. Engage the
abdominals to release pressure on
the lumbar spine.

Helpful Hints: Since the torque
on the knees is strong, this posture
is not recommended for anyone
with knee injuries. If one cannot
sit upright with the feet outside
the hips, and the sit bones on the
ground, it is not recommended
to recline. To practice, try a half
Supta Virasana, or one leg at a
time. Do this toward the end of
class.

Counter Pose: *Baddha Konasana*
(see above, under "Pectineus")

Hip Inward Rotators

The main muscles are the
gluteus medius (anterior
fibers), gluteus minimus, tensor
fasciae latae, semitendinosus,
semimembranosus, pectineus, and
gracilis. These muscles have other
primary actions at the hip joint and
have already been discussed earlier
in this chapter.

**Asanas that heavily use these
muscles in inward (medial)
rotation**
Strengthening: *Supta Virasana*
(Reclined Hero Pose). *Prasarita
Padottanasana.*
Stretching: *Utkata Konasana*
(Goddess Pose). *Padmasana.
Baddha Konasana.*

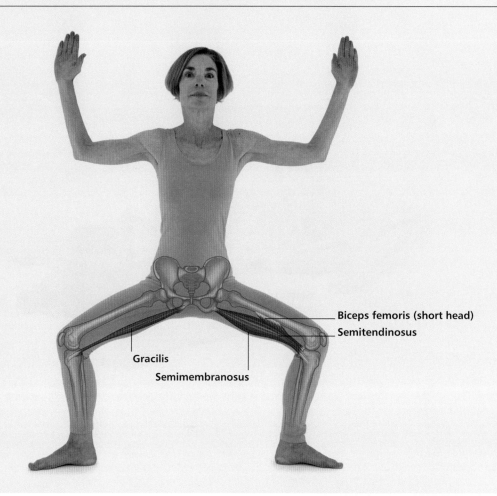

Biceps femoris (short head)
Semitendinosus
Gracilis
Semimembranosus

utkata = fierce, powerful; *kona* = angle; (oot-kah-tuh cone-AHS-anna)

Awareness: Breath, strength, stretch, power, core engagement, chest and hip opener, energizing, balance, concentration, stimulation of circulatory system and breathing.

Action and Alignment: Spine extension, shoulder girdle stabilization, shoulder joint abduction, hip flexion and outward rotation, knee flexion. Body is in line from the mid-ear to the hip, with the knees over the toes.

Technique: From *Tadasana* facing the long side of the mat, stand with the legs three feet apart. Turn the legs out to a 45-degree angle, and bend the knees out over the toes. Engage the pelvic floor and abdominals, and drop the tailbone. One can add bandha work here as well. The position of the arms can vary—the Cactus (shown) and prayer positions are common. For more of a challenge, raise the arms high while pressing the shoulders down. This pose is strength work for the hip flexors and outward rotators, and stretch for the hip extensors and inward rotators, as well as stabilization for the adductors and abductors—a great asana for the hips!

Helpful Hints: This is a squat position and therefore an intense strength pose for the lower extremity. The longer the pose is held, the higher the level achieved. Try one to two minutes, without losing the alignment or breath. It is said to be excellent for pregnant women; try it against the wall for support. Tap into the Goddess within whether male or female. The posture can be done at any time during class when power and stability are needed.

Counter Pose: *Tadasana.*

Virabhadrasana III (Warrior III) Level II (Summary Pose)

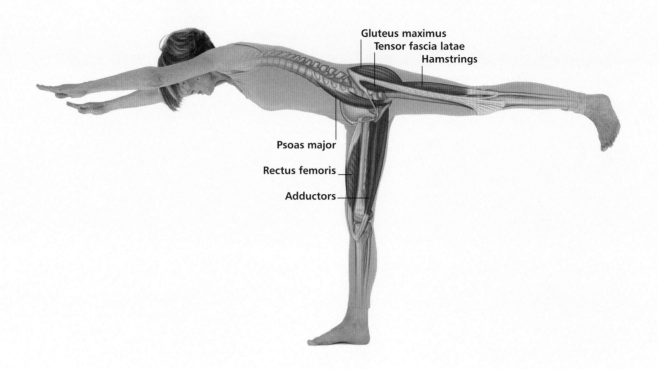

Gluteus maximus
Tensor fascia latae
Hamstrings

Psoas major

Rectus femoris

Adductors

Virabhadra = warrior or super-being from Indian mythology; (veer-ah-bah-DRAHS-anna)

Awareness: Breath, strength, stretch, core engagement, balance, concentration.

Action and Alignment: Spine extension, shoulder girdle stabilization, abduction and adduction (secondary)shoulder joint flexion, hip flexion and extension, knee extension, ankle dorsiflexion or plantar flexion. Body is in a straight horizontal line, with balance over the standing leg.

Technique: From *Tadasana* to *Virabhadrasana I*, lean the upper body forward into a diagonal line with the back leg. Reaching either forward or onto blocks, begin to straighten the front knee as the back leg lifts off the ground. Assume a horizontal line from the back of the head, through the arms to the back leg, parallel to the floor. Different arm positions can be used: arms reaching forward, reaching back, or in prayer position are some variations.

Helpful Hints: If using blocks, place them on the outside of each foot before beginning the pose. When in the asana, make sure the back leg is neutral at the hip, with the knee and foot facing down. Hold the posture for at least three full breaths. *Virabhadrasana III* can be done during class after the core has been warmed up. Remember, the core is the key to all standing and one-leg balances.

Counter Pose: *Tadasana*.

9 Muscles of the Knee

The knee is a highly specialized design mechanism. It is supposedly the largest joint in the body, with the two long bones (femur and tibia) acting as levers. Where they meet there is good sagittal movement, but little lateral movement. This fact, plus the location of the knee between the hip and the foot, makes it vulnerable to injury. Yoga, with correct attention to postural alignment, can keep the knees healthy and strong.

Structure

The femur (thigh bone) is the heaviest bone in the body. It articulates with the concave surface of the tibia to create the main composition of the knee. Add the patella (kneecap) as protection, and the fibula bone as an anchor for tendons and ligaments, and the structure becomes more efficient.

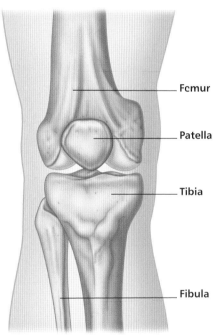

Bones of the knee, right leg, anterior view.

Connective Tissue

Because of the knee's exposure, its ligaments and tendons must be in good working order to maintain integrity of the structure. On each side of the knee there is a collateral ligament: the tibial (medial) collateral ligament on the inside and the fibular (lateral) collateral ligament on the outside. The anterior and posterior cruciate ligaments cross inside the knee joint. Cartilage (the medial and lateral menisci) lies between the two main bones, with hyaline cartilage behind the patella for cushioning. The patellar ligament keeps the kneecap in place, joining with the quadriceps tendon to attach to the front of the tibia. There are bursae around the joint area to reduce friction.

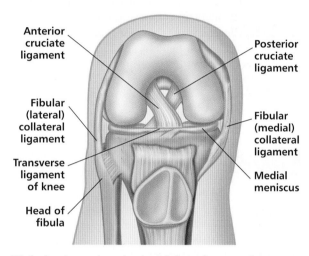

Right leg (anterior view) with knee bent at ninety degrees.

Labels:
- Anterior cruciate ligament
- Posterior cruciate ligament
- Fibular (lateral) collateral ligament
- Fibular (medial) collateral ligament
- Transverse ligament of knee
- Medial meniscus
- Head of fibula

Actions

The knee's primary actions are flexion (knee bending) and extension (knee straightening). Little known but of great importance is its secondary action in the horizontal plane—inward and outward rotation. This can only happen when the knee is bent (flexed), and the action aids in correct tibial traction.

Muscles

The quadriceps muscles, at the front of the upper leg, are the main extensors, and active in many movements—such as walking, running, jumping, and kicking—and in any movement that straightens the knee. These muscles form the most powerful and largest muscle group in the human body. They are stronger than their antagonists, the hamstrings. It is desirable to have the quadriceps at least 25% stronger than the hamstrings in order to balance the mechanisms of the knee joint.

The hamstrings, at the back of the upper leg, are the main flexors, with other biarticulate muscles from the hip sharing the load (such as the sartorius and gracilis—see Chapter 8). The short popliteus is also posterior and invaluable in checking knee hyperextension.

Knee Flexors

Primary muscles: biceps femoris, semitendinosus, semimembranosus (see "Hamstrings," Chapter 8).

Secondary muscles: sartorius, gracilis (see Chapter 8); gastrocnemius (see Chapter 10).

Knee Outward Rotators (Knee Flexed)

Biceps femoris (see "Hamstrings," Chapter 8), vastus lateralis (see above, under "Quadriceps").

For asanas, see *Supta Virasana* (Chapter 8, under "Hip Inward Rotators"). The thighs will rotate in, but the knees actually rotate out.

Knee Inward Rotators (Knee Flexed)

Semitendinosus, semimembranosus, sartorius, gracilis, vastus medialis (see Chapter 8, as well as under "Quadriceps" above).

There is actually no asana that is ideal for inward rotation of the knee. See *Prasarita Padottanasana* (Wide-leg Forward Bend, Chapter 4.) If the knees are flexed, the lower legs can rotate in. The muscles (listed above) that do this action can be worked in other ways, since most are biarticulate or can also do knee flexion or extension.

QUADRICEPS (KNEE EXTENSORS)

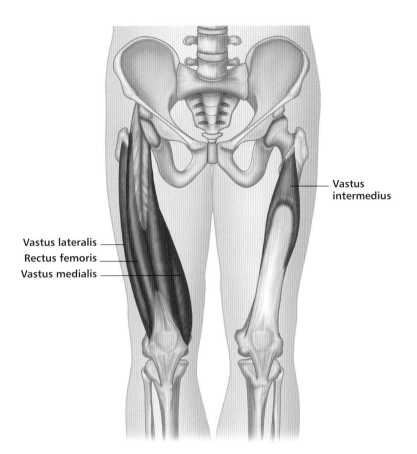

Vastus intermedius

Vastus lateralis

Rectus femoris

Vastus medialis

Latin, *quadriceps*, four-headed.

The four quadriceps muscles are the rectus femoris (see Chapter 8), the vastus lateralis, vastus medialis, and vastus intermedius. All these muscles cross the knee joint, but the rectus femoris is the only one that has two heads of origin and that also crosses the hip joint (where it causes flexion). The quadriceps muscles straighten the knee when rising from sitting, during walking, and while climbing. As a group, the vasti muscles aid, by eccentric contraction, in controlling the movement of sitting down.

Origin
Rectus femoris: Front part of ilium (anterior inferior iliac spine). Area above hip socket.
Vasti: Upper half of shaft of femur.

Insertion
Patella, then via patellar ligament into the upper anterior part of the tibia (tibial tuberosity).

Action
Rectus femoris: Extends the knee joint and flexes the hip joint (particularly in combination, as in kicking a ball).
Vasti: Extends the knee joint.
Note: the portion of the medial vastus muscle that is just above the knee is sometimes referred to as the "vastus medialis obliquus," or VMO, which is activated with full extension.

Nerve
Femoral nerve, L2, L3, L4.

Basic functional movement
Example: Walking up stairs. Cycling.

Movements that may injure these muscles
Running, jumping, squats with heavy weight.

Common problems when muscles are chronically tight/ shortened
Knee pain, knee instability, especially if tight and weak.

Asanas that heavily use these muscles
Strengthening: All One-leg Balances; *Utkatasana* (Chair) for rectus femoris in hip flexion, all quadriceps strengthen on return. *Uttanasana. Adho Mukha Svanasana, Urdhva Mukha Svanasana. Virabhadrasanas I, II, III* (back leg). *Trikonasana. Natarajasana* (supporting leg). *Vrksasana* (supporting leg).
Stretching: *Janu Sirsasana* (bent leg). *Ustrasana. Supta Virasana. Natarajasana* (non-supporting leg). *Vrksasana* (non-supporting leg). *Natarajasana* is mentioned as a stretch for the back leg because both ends of the muscle (tendons) are lengthened when the hip is extended and the knee is flexed. Here is a good example of isometric contraction as a strengthening move also: while the foot is pressed into the hand, strap or wall, the muscle is working against an immoveable force. The bottom leg is doing the same: isometrically contracting.

Natarajasana (Lord of the Dance Pose) Level I

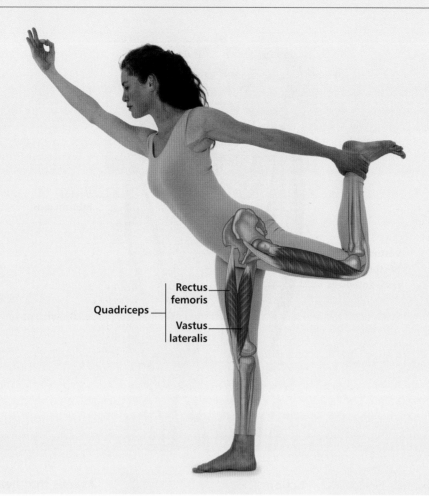

Quadriceps

Rectus femoris

Vastus lateralis

nata = dancer; *raja* = king; (nat-tah-raj-AHS-anna)

Awareness: Breath, strength, anterior stretch, hip and chest opener, balance, concentration.

Action and Alignment: Spine extension to hyperextension, shoulder girdle forward tilt (back arm), shoulder joint hyperextension (back arm), hip and knee flexion and extension, ankle dorsiflexion. The body remains upright with the pelvis centered.

Technique: From *Tadasana*, shift the weight to one leg. Bend the other knee and reach back for the ankle. Pushing that foot into the hand, begin to raise the free leg as the pelvis tilts slightly. Counter the balance with the free hand reaching forward. It is very important to lift the core here, as the belly will tend to hang. The gaze and chest are forward.

Helpful Hints: Use a wall for support with the free hand. A strap placed around the foot and held with both hands is also good; the arms and strap are lifted up behind the head. This pose can be done at any time after the hips and lumbar spine have been warmed up.

Counter Pose: Repeat on the other side, then do *Adho Mukha Svanasana*.

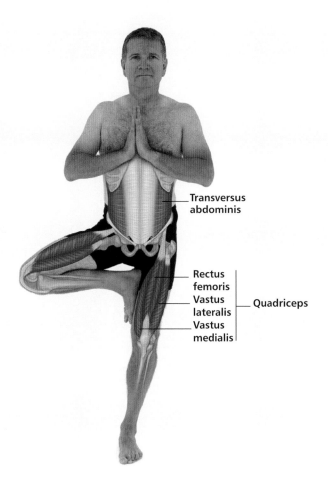

Transversus
abdominis

Rectus
femoris

Vastus
lateralis

Vastus
medialis

Quadriceps

vrksa = tree; (vrik-SHAHS-anna)

Awareness: Breath, strength, stretch, hip opener, core, balance, energy, concentration.

Action and Alignment: Spine extension, shoulder stabilization, hip flexion and outward rotation (free leg), knee flexion and extension. The body is in full upright alignment, with the shoulders and pelvis even.

Technique: From *Tadasana*, bring the weight evenly over one foot without shifting the hips (use the core to accomplish this). Raise the other leg, using the hand to help place the sole of the foot either above or below the knee on the inside of the standing leg. Open the hip of the top leg to an outwardly rotated position, without turning or lifting the pelvis. Drop the tailbone, lift the pelvic floor, and place the hands in prayer position. The gaze is forward or up.

Helpful Hints: Counterbalance the foot and leg against one another. Think of the bottom leg rooted to the ground. If balance is achieved, raise the arms toward the sky, pressing the shoulders down away from the ears. Use a wall or chair support if necessary. This pose can be done at any time after the hips have been warmed up.

Counter Pose: *Tadasana*, then do the other side.

POPLITEUS

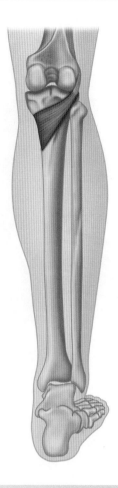

Latin, *poples*, the ham.

A small diagonal muscle behind the knee and mainly a stabilizer. The tendon from the origin of popliteus lies inside the capsule of the knee joint.

Origin
Lateral surface of lateral condyle of femur. Oblique popliteal ligament of knee joint.

Insertion
Upper part of posterior surface of tibia, superior to soleal line.

Action
Laterally rotates femur on tibia when foot is fixed on the ground. Medially rotates tibia on femur when the leg is non-weight-bearing. Assists flexion of knee joint (popliteus "unlocks" the extended knee joint to initiate flexion of the leg). Helps reinforce posterior ligaments of knee joint.

Nerve
Tibial nerve, L4, L5, S1.

Basic functional movement
Example: Walking.

Movements that may injure these muscles
Hyperextension of the knee. Jumping/landing. Squats with heavy weight.

Common problems when muscles are chronically tight/shortened
Knee pain, knee instability, especially if weak.

Asanas that heavily use these muscles
Strengthening: *Utkatasana. Virabhadrasanas I, II* (front leg). *Alanasana* (front leg).
Stretching: *Janu Sirsasana* (straight leg). *Adho Mukha Svanasana. Paschimottanasana.*

Utkatasana (Chair Pose) is used to demonstrate the hamstrings in a variety of ways. As knee flexors, these muscles are contracting isometrically to hold both knees in flexion, although on the way back up from the position the quadriceps will contract concentrically to straighten the knees against gravity and body weight, which are the main resistive forces. The hamstrings will contract concentrically on the way back up from sitting, working as hip extensors (remember they are biarticulate). *Utkatasana* is a deep hip and knee flexion position, but the main work is in the holding, and the moving back up.

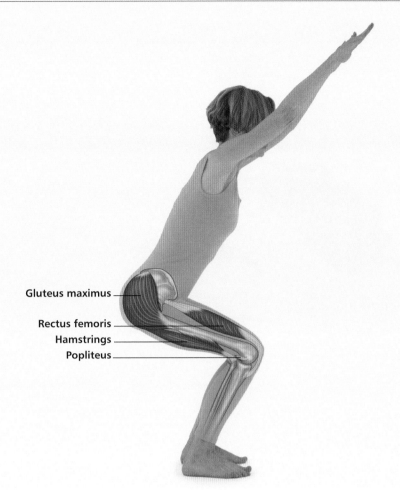

Gluteus maximus
Rectus femoris
Hamstrings
Popliteus

utkata = powerful; (oot-kah-TAHS-anna)

Awareness: Breath, strength, stretch, chest expansion, core support, stimulation of organs.

Action and Alignment: Spine extension, shoulder girdle stabilization, shoulder joint flexion, hip flexion to extension and adduction, knee flexion to extension, ankle dorsiflexion. Body is in a straight line from the arms to the ear to the hip.

Technique: From *Tadasana*, deeply bend the knees as if sitting in a chair. The spine is straight as the arms are raised up in line with the ears. The gaze is forward or up, and the chest is forward. This is a difficult movement: the core must work strongly to keep the belly and the pelvic floor lifted, as the tailbone drops. Ideally the thighs become parallel to the ground.

Helpful Hints: Care must be taken not to increase the curvature of the lumbar spine. The hands can be placed on the hips, or a Cactus arm position adopted, to aid if there are any shoulder issues. The posture is held for a minute, and can be done at any time during class. It is a part of *Surya Namaskar B* (Sun Salutation B).

Counter Pose: *Tadasana* with a backward stretch.

Paschimottanasana (Sitting Forward Bend) Level I (Knee Flexor Stretch)

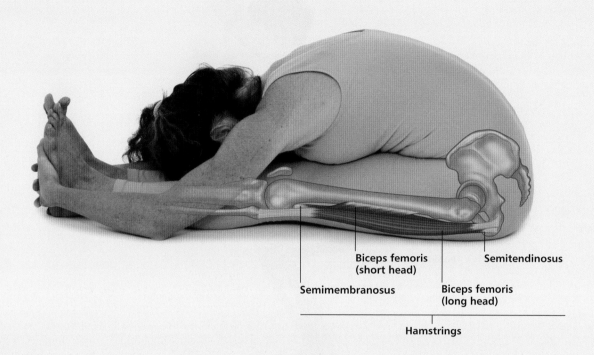

Biceps femoris (short head)

Semitendinosus

Semimembranosus

Biceps femoris (long head)

Hamstrings

pascha = west, back; *uttana* = intense stretch; (pash-ee-moh-tan-AHS-anna)

Awareness: Breath, posterior stretch, spine, hip and leg flexibility, stimulation of organs, digestion, calming.

Action and Alignment: Spine extension, shoulder stabilization, hip flexion, knee extension, ankle dorsiflexion. Body is in a straight line from the head to the hips.

Technique: From a sitting position, extend both legs out in front while sitting straight up. Hinge forward from the hips, lifting the pelvis up and over the legs. The arms can reach forward, as long as the spine is not compromised. Ideally both knees and the spine are straight, with the toes pointing up.

Helpful Hints: If the hamstrings are tight, bend the knees or place a blanket underneath. One can also sit on a block or blanket. Once the extended spine position is reached, the spine can flex forward, as demonstrated in the image. This posture is best done toward the end of class, when the body is warm.

Counter Pose: *Ardha Purvottanasana* (see Chapter 6).

10 Muscles of the Lower Leg and Foot

The lower leg and foot support all the structures above them, and this is not an easy task. The arch-like construction of the foot (ankle and toe joints) allows it to perform the functions of support, adaptability, shock absorption, weight transfer, and propulsion. In yoga, the feet are the foundation of many asanas.

Structure

There are 26 bones, 19 large muscles, many small intrinsic muscles on the sole of the foot, and over 100 ligaments that together constitute the main structure of *each* lower leg/foot. The transfer of weight from the tibia to the talus, and then to the calcaneus (heel bone), is an amazing balancing act as the weight of the entire body is accepted and then propelled forward through the rest of the foot.

The arches are a lesson in architecture. Three arches form a "dome" to perform the necessary functions of the foot. The main longitudinal arch is on the medial side, consisting of the calcaneus on one side and four tarsals on the front, with the talus in the middle acting as the "keystone." Laterally a longitudinal arch travels from the calcaneus through the talus to the cuboid and fourth and fifth metatarsals. The transverse arch crosses the foot from the big toe to the little toe metatarsal. The action of all the lines of force is centered where the transverse and longitudinal arches meet, accepting body weight from above and ground impact from below. The extrinsic muscles of the foot and the muscles in the sole (intrinsic) reinforce the arches. Put the two feet together, parallel, and a complete dome is formed in the center of both: *Tadasana!*

Actions

At the upper ankle joint, there is plantar flexion (foot pointed) and dorsiflexion (foot flexed). The lower ankle pronates (a combination of eversion and abduction) and supinates (a combination of inversion and adduction). The toes mainly flex and extend; these actions help spread the toes, a desirable "feat" in yoga.

The muscles of the lower leg will be covered first.

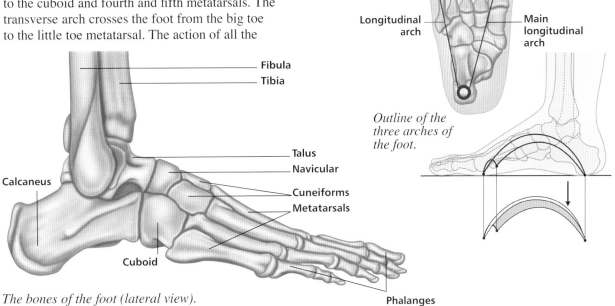

Outline of the three arches of the foot.

The bones of the foot (lateral view).

Labels: Fibula, Tibia, Talus, Navicular, Cuneiforms, Metatarsals, Calcaneus, Cuboid, Phalanges

Transverse arch, Longitudinal arch, Main longitudinal arch

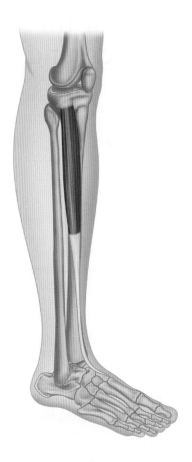

Latin, *tibialis*, relating to the shin; *anterior*, in front.

Origin
Lateral condyle of tibia. Upper half of lateral surface of tibia. Interosseous membrane.

Insertion
Medial and plantar surface of medial cuneiform bone. Base of first metatarsal.

Action
Dorsiflexes ankle joint. Inverts ankle joint.

Nerve
Deep peroneal nerve, L4, L5, S1.

Basic functional movement
Example: Walking and running (helps prevent the foot from slapping onto the ground after the heel strikes, and lifts the foot clear of the ground as the leg swings forward).

EXTENSOR DIGITORUM LONGUS

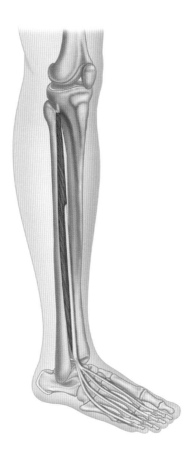

Latin, *extendere*, to extend; *digitus*, finger/toe; *longus*, long.

Like the corresponding tendons in the hand, this muscle forms extensor hoods on the dorsum of the proximal phalanges of the foot. These hoods are joined by the tendons of the lumbricales and extensor digitorum brevis, but not by the interossei.

Origin
Lateral condyle of tibia. Upper two-thirds of anterior surface of fibula. Upper part of interosseous membrane.

Insertion
Along dorsal surface of the four lateral toes. Each tendon divides to attach to the bases of the middle and distal phalanges.

Action
Extends toes at the metatarsophalangeal joints. Assists extension of the interphalangeal joints. Assists dorsiflexion of the ankle joint and eversion of the foot.

Nerve
Fibular (peroneal) nerve, L4, L5, S1.

Basic functional movement
Example: Walking up stairs (ensuring the toes clear the steps).

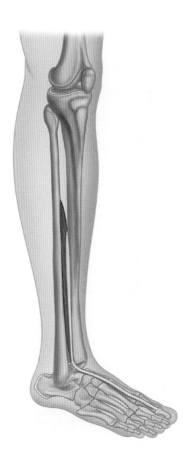

Latin, *extendere*, to extend; *hallux*, big toe; *longus*, long.

This muscle lies between and deep to tibialis anterior and extensor digitorum longus.

Origin
Middle half of anterior surface of fibula and adjacent interosseous membrane.

Insertion
Base of distal phalanx of great toe.

Action
Extends all the joints of the big toe. Dorsiflexes the ankle joint. Assists inversion of the foot.

Nerve
Deep fibular (peroneal) nerve, L4, L5, S1.

Basic functional movement
Example: Walking up stairs (ensuring the big toe clears the steps).

This position of the foot is used in many asanas (e.g. *Janu Sirsasana*), strengthening the front of the lower leg and stretching the posterior portion.

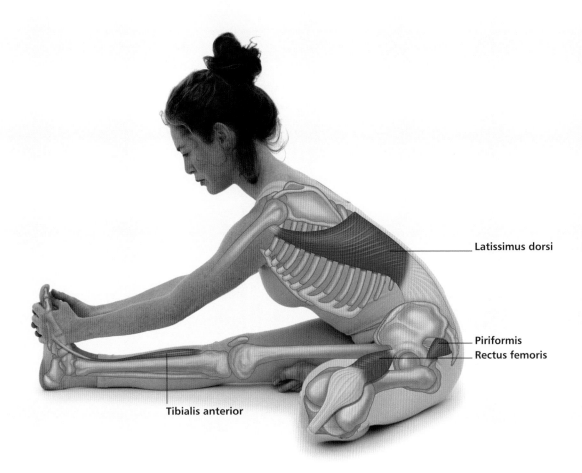

Latissimus dorsi

Piriformis
Rectus femoris

Tibialis anterior

janu = knee; *sirsa* = head; (jahn-u shear-SHAHS-anna)

Awareness: Breath, stretch, stimulates organs, therapeutic, calming.

Action and Alignment: Spine extension, shoulder girdle stabilization, shoulder joint flexion, hip and knee flexion and extension, ankle dorsiflexion. Body is in straight line from the head to the hips.

Technique: From a sitting position, extend one leg in front and bend the opposite leg, placing that foot on the inside of the other thigh. Keeping the spine straight, hinge at the hips and reach forward with the hands, placing them on the straight leg. Anchor the sit bones and engage the core. Hold the posture and breathe deeply.

Helpful Hints: Relax the straight knee if the hamstrings are too tight. Keep the chest and shoulders square toward the front leg. Sit on a blanket for support. Once the position has been accomplished, the spine can flex, bringing the head toward the knee. This posture can be done at any time during class, and is considered a warm-up for *Paschimottanasana* (Sitting Forward Bend) with both legs straight.

Counter Pose: Reverse Plank.

TIBIALIS POSTERIOR

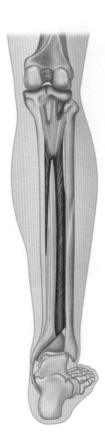

Latin, *tibialis*, relating to the shin; *posterior*, behind.

Tibialis posterior is the deepest muscle on the back of the leg. It helps maintain the arches of the foot.

Origin
Lateral part of posterior surface of tibia. Upper two-thirds of posterior surface of fibula. Most of interosseous membrane.

Insertion
Tuberosity of navicular. By fibrous expansions to the sustentaculum tali, three cuneiforms, and cuboid and bases of the second, third, and fourth metatarsals.

Action
Inverts ankle joint. Assists in plantar flexion of ankle joint.

Nerve
Tibial nerve, L4, L5, S1.

Basic functional movement
Examples: Standing on tiptoes. Pushing down car pedals.

FIBULARIS (PERONEUS) TERTIUS

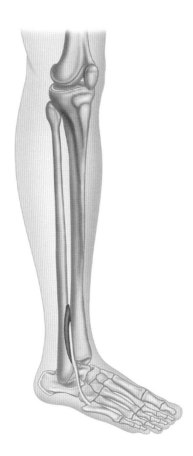

Latin, *fibula*, pin/buckle; *tertius*, third. **Greek**, *perone*, pin/buckle.

This muscle is a partially separated, lower lateral part of extensor digitorum longus.

Origin
Lower third of anterior surface of fibula and interosseous membrane.

Insertion
Dorsal surface of base of fifth metatarsal.

Action
Dorsiflexes ankle joint. Everts ankle joint.

Nerve
Deep fibular (peroneal) nerve, L4, L5, S1.

Basic functional movement
Examples: Walking and running.

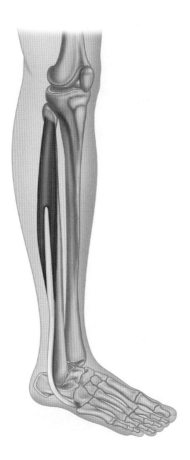

Latin, *fibula*, pin/buckle; *longus*, long. **Greek**, *perone*, pin/buckle.

The course of the tendon of insertion of fibularis longus helps maintain the transverse and lateral longitudinal arches of the foot.

Origin
Upper two-thirds of lateral surface of fibula. Lateral condyle of tibia.

Insertion
Lateral side of medial cuneiform. Base of first metatarsal.

Action
Everts ankle joint. Assists plantar flexion of ankle joint.

Nerve
Superficial fibular (peroneal) nerve, L4, L5, S1.

Basic functional movement
Example: Walking on uneven surfaces.

FIBULARIS (PERONEUS) BREVIS

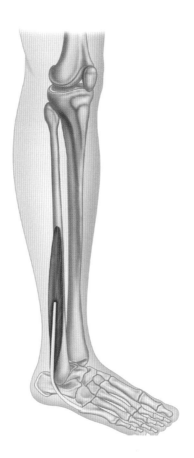

Latin, *fibula*, pin/buckle; *brevis*, short. **Greek**, *perone*, pin/buckle.

A slip of muscle from fibularis brevis often joins the long extensor tendon of the little toe, whereupon it is known as "peroneus digiti minimi."

Origin
Lower two-thirds of lateral surface of fibula. Adjacent intermuscular septa.

Insertion
Lateral side of base of fifth metatarsal.

Action
Everts ankle joint. Assists plantar flexion of ankle joint.

Nerve
Superficial fibular (peroneal) nerve, L4, L5, S1.

Basic functional movement
Example: Walking on uneven ground.

GASTROCNEMIUS

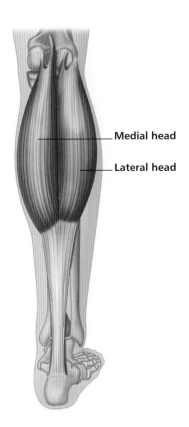

Medial head
Lateral head

Greek, *gaster*, stomach; *kneme*, lower leg.

Gastrocnemius is part of the composite muscle known as "triceps surae," which forms the prominent contour of the calf. The triceps surae comprises the gastrocnemius, soleus, and plantaris. The popliteal fossa at the back of the knee is formed inferiorly by the bellies of gastrocnemius and plantaris, laterally by the tendon of biceps femoris, and medially by the tendons of semimembranosus and semitendinosus.

Origin
Medial head: Popliteal surface of femur, above medial condyle.
Lateral head: Lateral condyle and posterior surface of femur.

Insertion
Posterior surface of calcaneus (via the tendo calcaneus, which is a fusion of the tendons of gastrocnemius and soleus).

Action
Plantar flexes foot at ankle joint. Assists in flexion of knee joint. It is a main propelling force in walking and running.

Nerve
Tibial nerve, S1, S2.

Basic functional movement
Example: Standing on tiptoes.

SOLEUS

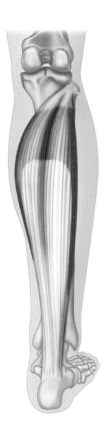

Latin, *solea*, leather sole/sandal/sole (fish).

Soleus is part of the triceps surae and is so named because of its shape. The Achilles (calcaneal tendon) of the soleus and gastrocnemius is the thickest and strongest tendon in the body.

Origin
Posterior surfaces of head of fibula and upper third of body of fibula. Soleal line and middle third of medial border of tibia. Tendinous arch between tibia and fibula.

Insertion
With tendon of gastrocnemius into posterior surface of calcaneus.

Action
Plantar flexes ankle joint. The soleus is frequently in contraction during standing to prevent the body falling forward at the ankle joint (i.e., to offset the line of pull through the body's center of gravity). Thus it helps to maintain an upright posture.

Nerve
Tibial nerve, L5, S1, S2.

Basic functional movement
Example: Standing on the balls of the feet.

Utkatasana has already been described in Chapter 9 as a hamstring exercise. The illustration shown here is a variation with the toes raised, which incorporates plantar flexion of the ankle joint.

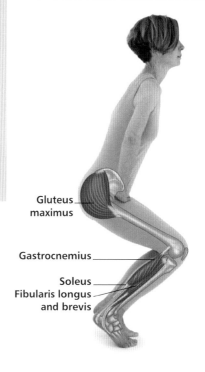

Gluteus maximus

Gastrocnemius

Soleus
Fibularis longus and brevis

Foot

The feet are considered the foundation of most yoga asanas. Beginning with *Tadasana* (Mountain Pose) as an initial point, the feet are "grounded" through what are called "the four corners of the foot." Students are asked to become aware of where the weight is being held, and to balance with the toes forward in a parallel position (heels behind toes). The toes are also cued to "spread" (abduction). Once this is experienced, the alignment process travels up through the legs, the pelvis, and the spine in an active manner in order to initiate length, space, and prana up through the body. Feeling the connection to the earth, through the feet, and up and out to the universe is an example of the energetic quality and health benefits of yoga.

The muscles of the foot are listed here and can be referenced in more detail in other sources if needed. Keep in mind there are three main areas: (1) the upper ankle joint, where dorsiflexion and plantar flexion occur; (2) the lower ankle joint, with joint actions of pronation and supination; and (3) the phalanges (toes), with flexion, extension, abduction, and adduction (similar to the fingers). Some of the muscles are multiarticulate, working two or more joints, and have been discussed above in the "Lower Leg" section.

Metatarsophalangeal Joints
Plantar and dorsal interossei muscles (abduct and flex)

Foot Muscles

Intrinsic (sole of foot) and Extrinsic (dorsal side)
Hallucis (big toe) muscles: Abductor hallucis, abductor digiti minimi (pinky toe), flexor hallucis brevis, flexor hallucis longus, adductor hallucis, extensor hallucis longus

Toe Flexors
Flexor digitorum brevis, flexor digitorum longus, flexor digiti minimi brevis, quadratus plantae, lumbricales (flex metatarsophalangeal joints)

Toe Extensors
Lumbricales (lateral side toe extension), interossei, extensor digitorum brevis

Toe Abductors
Dorsal interossei

Toe Adductors
Plantar interossei

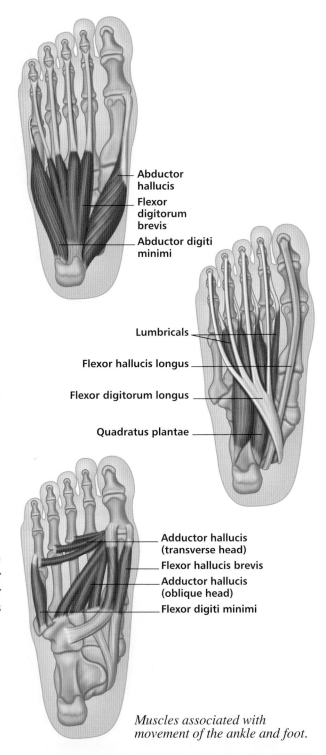

- Abductor hallucis
- Flexor digitorum brevis
- Abductor digiti minimi

- Lumbricals
- Flexor hallucis longus
- Flexor digitorum longus
- Quadratus plantae

- Adductor hallucis (transverse head)
- Flexor hallucis brevis
- Adductor hallucis (oblique head)
- Flexor digiti minimi

Muscles associated with movement of the ankle and foot.

Basic functional movement
Facilitate walking.

Movements that may injure these muscles
Misalignment. Irritation of plantar fascia (superficial tissue, similar to "padding"). Incorrect walking pattern/shoes.

Asanas that heavily use these muscles
All asanas that use grounding of the foot, dorsiflexion, or plantar flexion.

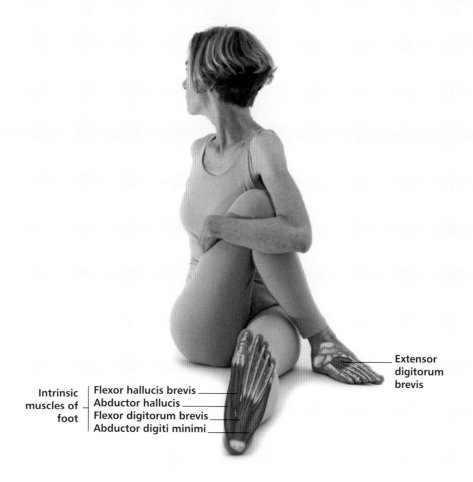

Extensor digitorum brevis

Intrinsic muscles of foot
- Flexor hallucis brevis
- Abductor hallucis
- Flexor digitorum brevis
- Abductor digiti minimi

ardha = half; *matsya* = fish; *Indra* = ruler; (Ar-dah mot-see-en-DRAHS-anna)

Awareness: Breath, stretch, strength, release, stimulation of organs, energizing.

Action and Alignment: Spine extension and rotation, shoulder stabilization, hip flexion and adduction, knee flexion and extension, ankle dorsiflexion and plantar flexion. Most important alignment is full spinal extension, with the weight on top of the sit bones.

Technique: From a sitting position, extend one leg forward and place the other foot on the inside or outside of the bottom leg. Extend the spine and begin to rotate toward the bent knee side, using the hand or elbow as an anchor against the leg. Begin the twist from the thoracic through the cervical spine, inhaling to extend and exhaling to deepen the twist.

Helpful Hints: For more of a challenge, fold the bottom leg underneath. Hold and deepen for three full breaths before returning to center. Repeat on the other side. This twist can be done at any time during class, as long as the spine and hips have been active.

Counter Pose: *Paschimottanasana* (see Chapter 9): then a supine half-bridge.

Appendix 1: Final Poses

Final pose descriptions and illustrations are placed here, completing the collection of asanas that are usually required for a 200-hour Level I yoga teacher training course.

The first is *Sarvangasana* (Shoulder Stand Pose)— "The Queen of Asanas".

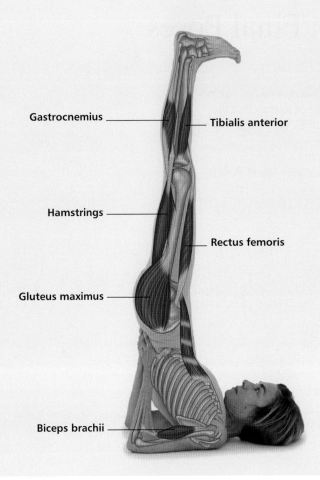

Gastrocnemius

Tibialis anterior

Hamstrings

Rectus femoris

Gluteus maximus

Biceps brachii

sarva = all; *anga* = limbs; (sar-van-GAHS-anna)

Awareness: Breath, strength, stabilization, core, extension, inversion, harmony, increase in circulation and digestion, stimulation of PNS, organs, and thyroid/prostate glands, calming.

Action and Alignment: Spine extension, shoulder stabilization, core stabilization, hip neutral, knee extension, ankle dorsiflexion or plantar flexion. Body is in a straight vertical line.

Technique: There are a variety of ways to begin this posture, depending on the level (for Level I use the wall). Beginning on the mat, lie down in a supine position, with the knees bent and the feet flat on the floor. Lift the hips to *Setu Bandhasana* (Chapter 8) for a warm-up, placing the hands under the hips. The legs can kick up from here, or lying down flat one can roll into the inversion. Use the hands under the hips to help lift the torso and legs skyward, walking the shoulder blades together for support and balance, as this is where the weight is. The gaze is toward the chest. To come down, simply roll through the spine gently and slowly, with aid from the hands.

Helpful Hints: The most important recommendation is to place a folded blanket or two under the shoulders, allowing the neck to be free, with the head in line with the upper spine. Ideally the bottom tips of the shoulder blades are in a straight line with the heels. Even though an inversion of this type is so beneficial, there are contraindications, such as heavy menstrual flow, glaucoma and retinal eye conditions, pregnancy, and high blood pressure. If none of these conditions is present, the pose can be held from one to five minutes, and is done toward the end of class.

Counter Pose: *Matsyasana* (see Chapter 7) or *Bhujangasana* (see Chapter 4).

The following asana—Plow Pose—can be done before or after Shoulder Stand.

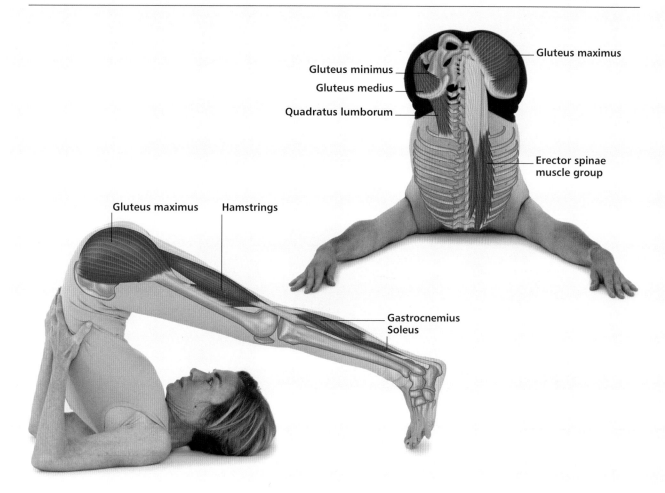

Gluteus minimus

Gluteus medius

Quadratus lumborum

Gluteus maximus

Erector spinae muscle group

Gluteus maximus   Hamstrings

Gastrocnemius Soleus

hala = plow; (hal-AHS-anna)

Awareness: Breath, stretch, inversion, stress relief, therapeutic, calming yet invigorating.

Action and Alignment: Spine extension, shoulder stabilization, hip flexion, knee extension, ankle dorsiflexion. Spine is straight, with the shoulders to the hips in a vertical line.

Technique: Either complete this posture from *Sarvangasana*, or roll into it from a sitting or lying down position, allowing the feet to come behind the head. Extend the legs, and support the pose with the balls of the feet into the ground. Use the cues from *Sarvangasana* to deepen the pose.

Helpful Hints: Many practitioners go into spine flexion in this posture, but it is best to try to lift the tailbone toward the sky, extending the spine. Be careful of the neck; if there are no problems in this region, one can extend the arms underneath, clasping the hands. Hold, and then return as one would from *Sarvangasana*.

Counter Pose: *Matsyasana* (see Chapter 7); *Adho Mukha Svanasana* (see Chapter 6).

A nice sequence to begin the cool-down at the end of class is: *Sarvangasana*, *Halasana*, *Matsyasana*, *Setu Bandhasana*, Knees to Chest, Supine Twist; Happy Baby; *Savasana*.

Every yoga class or practice ends with *Savasana*, described next—the "easiest to do, but hardest to master," as one simply lies down, and then surrenders.

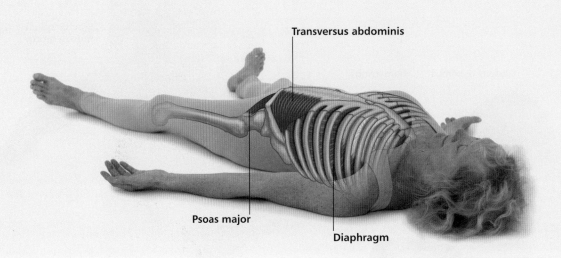

Transversus abdominis

Psoas major

Diaphragm

sava = corpse; (shah-VAHS-anna)

Awareness: Stillness, softness, rest.

Action and Alignment: Body is supported completely by the ground, giving into gravity.

Technique: Lie down in a supine position, with the legs slightly apart, allowing the weight of the thighs to roll outward naturally. The arms extend down with the palms facing up, not touching the body or any other prop. The head can rest on a blanket if desired. Let go of thoughts, emotions, and any tension.

Helpful Hints: As the body cools down, it is wise to cover oneself with a blanket; using an eye pillow is also helpful. There are many ways to guide one through *Savasana*, with the main purpose being relaxation and inner peace, without sleeping. After ten minutes, bring back awareness slowly, then curl into a fetal position for a final release, before sitting up gently, using the hands to help, and bringing the head up last.

Counter Pose: Sitting meditation.

Appendix 2: "Cueing" in Yoga Asanas

How many different ways can someone teach something so that students will understand? Keeping things simple and clear is the most effective approach, with occasional changes introduced to keep the instructions fresh. Anatomy can be a complex language for some, so using too many technical terms can be counterproductive.

The following are samples of cues that can be used while teaching yoga; some of them may work and some may not, but have fun trying them out.

Breathing

Inhale and expand.
Exhale and release.
Nourish the body with the inhale.
Cleanse the body with the exhale.

Cueing the Spine

Drop (*not* "tuck"!) the tailbone.
Find your neutral (natural) curves.
Create space between the vertebrae.
Keep the head in line with the spine.
Keep the back of the skull in line with the back of the pelvis.
Allow the chin to relax in toward the throat, not the chest.
Imagine the head floating above the neck.

Cueing the Core

Lift the lower abdominals.
Pull the navel center in and up.
Feel the transversus abdominis wrap around the waistline on a strong exhale.
Do a deep belly laugh; the transversus will contract.
Lift or hug the pelvic floor.
Lengthen the lumbar spine.
Allow the belly to fall back toward the spine.
Feel space between the hips and the ribs.

Cueing the Shoulders

Drop the shoulders down and back.
Create space between your neck and your shoulders.
Allow the shoulder blades to come closer together and down the back.
Keep the shoulders even.
Circle your arms.
Open the shoulders.
Relax the shoulders.

Cueing the Hips

Center or square the pelvis.
Circle the thighs to lubricate the joint.
Deepen the hip crease.
Open the hips.
Tilt the pelvis.
Lift up and out of the hips.
Imagine the pelvis and femurs as an arch.
Find the sit bones and sit right on top of them.

Cueing the Knees

Soften the backs of the knees.
Gently bend, or micro-bend.
Track knees over toes, not forward of them.
Be kind to the knees.

Cueing the Feet

Spread the feet.
Balance on the four corners of the feet.
Lift the arches.
Pull the toes back.
Open the toes.
Soften the feet.
Feel the pads (balls) of the feet.

Great Verbs!

Begin	Open	Engage	Allow
Soften	Extend	Lengthen	Fold
Imagine	Create	Find	Lift
Drop	Contract	Spread	Balance
Connect	Nourish	Tone	Press
Draw	Increase	Decrease	Bend
Change	Straighten	Strengthen	Stretch
Improve	Help	Deepen	Release
Relax	Expand	Transform	Choose
Search	Experiment	Play	Grow
Adjust	Wonder	Thank	Give
Receive	Quiet	Master	Guide
Share	Invite	Love	*Breathe!*

Bibliography

Anderson, S. and Sovik, R. 2007. *Yoga: Mastering the Basics*, Honesdale, PA: Himalayan Institute.

Calais-Germain, B. 2007. *Anatomy of Movement*, Vista, CA: Eastland Press.

Coulter, D.H. 2001. *Anatomy of Hatha Yoga*, Honesdale, PA: Body and Breath.

Devananda, Swami Omkari 2009. *Yoga in the Shambhava Tradition*, Summertown, TN: Healthy Living Publications.

Jarmey, C. 2006. *The Concise Book of Muscles*, Chichester, UK/Berkeley, CA: Lotus Publishing/North Atlantic Books.

Kaminoff, L. 2007. *Yoga Anatomy*, Champaign, IL: Human Kinetics.

Keil, D. 2014. *Functional Anatomy of Yoga*, Chichester, UK: Lotus Publishing.

Lasater, J. 2009. *Yogabody: Anatomy, Kinesiology, and Asana*, Berkeley, CA: Rodmell Press.

Long, R. 2009. *The Key Muscles of Yoga*, Baldwinsville, NY: Bandha Yoga Publications.

Silva, M. and Shyam, M. 1997. *Yoga the Iyengar Way*, New York: Knopf.

Staugaard-Jones, J.A. 2010. *The Anatomy of Exercise & Movement: For the Study of Dance, Pilates, Sport and Yoga*, Chichester, UK: Lotus Publishing.

Staugaard-Jones, J.A. 2012. *The Vital Psoas Muscle*, Chichester, UK/Berkeley, CA: Lotus Publishing/North Atlantic Books.

Tigunait, P. R. 2014. *The Secret of the Yoga Sutra*. Himalayan Institute, 2014.

Index of Asanas

Sanskrit

Translation

Index of Muscles

Ordered by function/body region

Ordered alphabetically